A SHORT INTRODUCTION TO
PSYCHIATRY

Short Introductions to the Therapy Professions
Series Editor: Colin Feltham

Books in this series examine the different professions which provide help for people experiencing emotional or psychological problems. Written by leading practitioners and trainers in each field, the books are a source of up-to-date information about

- the nature of the work
- training, continuing professional development and career pathways
- the structure and development of the profession
- client populations and consumer views
- research and debates surrounding the profession.

Short Introductions to the Therapy Professions are ideal for anyone thinking about a career in one of the therapy professions or in the early stages of training. The books will also be of interest to mental health professionals needing to understand allied professions and also to patients, clients and relatives of service users.

Books in the series:

A Short Introduction to Clinical Psychology
Katherine Cheshire and David Pilgrim

A Short Introduction to Psychoanalysis
Jane Milton, Caroline Polmear and Julia Fabricius

A Short Introduction to Psychiatry
Linda Gask

A SHORT INTRODUCTION TO
PSYCHIATRY

Linda Gask

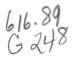 **SAGE** Publications
London ● Thousand Oaks ● New Delhi

SAGE Publications Ltd
1 Oliver's Yard
55 City Road
London EC1Y 1SP

SAGE Publications Inc.
2455 Teller Road
Thousand Oaks, California 91320

SAGE Publications India Pvt Ltd
B-42, Panchsheel Enclave
Post Box 4109
New Delhi 110 017

British Library Cataloguing in Publication data

A catalogue record for this book is available
from the British Library

ISBN 0 7619 7138 6
ISBN 0 7619 7139 4 (pbk)

Library of Congress Control Number: 2004102657

Typeset by C&M Digitals (P) Ltd, Chennai, India
Printed in Great Britain by TJ International Ltd, Padstow, Cornwall

**For my family, John and Suzy,
with all my love**

One need not be a Chamber to be Haunted
One need not be a House
The Brain has Corridors surpassing
Material Place

Emily Dickinson

CONTENTS

ACKNOWLEDGEMENTS

Several friends and colleagues kindly agreed to be interviewed and/or read early drafts of particular chapters and they are (in alphabetical order): Elaine Arnold, Tom Brown, Bill Deakin, Dinesh Bhugra, Chris Dowrick, Roger Farmer, Hugh Freeman, Chris Manning, Frank Margison, Max Marshall, Carl May, David Pilgrim, David Richards and Jenny Shaw. Mike Shooter, President of the Royal College of Psychiatrists gave up his precious time to talk to me. I also extend my thanks to the Royal College of Psychiatrists for giving me permission to reproduce material from their website in Appendix 1.

Colin Feltham suggested that I write the book and has been a very helpful editor, reading through drafts and posing some difficult questions. Finally I couldn't have completed this without my husband John, who always supports me even when I get carried away on yet another project.

INTRODUCTION

This book is not a textbook of psychiatry in the usual sense that a textbook generally contains the knowledge base of the subject in question. Instead it is a book *about* psychiatry, the profession and its practitioners, in the context of the history and culture of mental illness and mental health care. I hope that it will complement general textbooks of psychiatry and be of interest to psychiatrists in training, as well as to those considering psychiatry as a profession and other readers, including allied professionals, who simply want to understand what psychiatry *is*. Confusion often arises because 'psychiatry' may be used interchangeably with 'mental health care' and this book is concerned with the specific nature of the former as practised by psychiatrists rather than a broader examination of the provision of mental health care.

Johann Christian Reil (1759–1813), Professor of Medicine at Halle in Germany invented the term *psychiatry* at the turn of the nineteenth century. However, it was not until the early twentieth century that this began to be widely applied in English to a medical speciality. That psychiatry is indeed a speciality of medicine, a branch of medicine with its own training structure, sets it apart from the other mental health sciences and professions. But of all the branches of medicine, psychiatry sometimes seems to have the least connection with the school examinations in chemistry and biology that those who choose a medical career must take, and more in common with the social sciences.

In the past hundred years, people have turned increasingly to doctors when they have emotional problems. Psychiatrists have become the latest in a long line of people to manage the 'mad', following on from the magical healers and priests. But is there reason to think that psychiatrists deal better with such problems than anyone else? Today the person with religious delusions in the psychiatric unit can still see the priest and discuss his supposed sins, but the priest will probably suggest that he takes his medication too. However, the extent to which each psychiatrist will also explore the meaning of a particular symptom and how it might have arisen in that particular patient at that time in his or her life will vary considerably, depending on the weight he or she places on biology, psychodynamics and the social environment as aetiological and therapeutic factors in mental illness. The tensions between these three domains have been present to some degree throughout the history of psychiatry and form a central strand running throughout the chapters of this book, beginning in Chapter 1, which introduces psychiatry in its historical context.

Within psychiatry there has been confusion and even violent disagreement about what constitutes mental illness, what is required for a particular diagnosis and how different problems should be most effectively treated. Thomas Szasz, Professor of Psychiatry at Syracuse University, not only famously denied that there was any such thing as mental illness but further stated that:

> Psychiatry is conventionally defined as a medical specialty concerned with the diagnosis and treatment of mental diseases. I submit that this definition, which is still widely accepted, places psychiatry in the company of alchemy and astrology and commits it to the category of pseudo-science. (1974: 1–2)

Chapter 2 attempts to explore the culture of current psychiatric practice, how it is taught and what a psychiatrist actually does in his or her everyday work, in the context of the biological revolution that is now occurring in our understanding of mental illness.

To practise psychiatry, you have to be a doctor. Yet, unlike other medical specialities, psychiatry also has opponents within the profession who call themselves 'anti-psychiatrists', and even has practitioners who call themselves 'post-psychiatrists'. The question that many both outside and inside the profession are now asking is 'Is psychiatry trying to be too scientific?' Even Nancy Andreasen (2001), one of the leading proponents of biological psychiatry, thinks that the pendulum has shifted too far towards the biological. But she does not necessarily blame the new technology that has allowed us to visualize the brain and begin to understand the biological basis of mental illness. Instead, she cites the economic changes in the health-care system which make it too expensive for psychiatrists to spend their time doing psychotherapy, and excessive 'DSMism'– by which she means the all-pervading influence, on the way in which psychiatrists worldwide practise, of the *Diagnostic and Statistical Manual* of the American Psychiatric Association. Chapter 3 explores how the professional work of psychiatry is currently experienced, by psychiatrists in practice, our fellow mental health professionals and our patients.

From an entirely different viewpoint, Arthur Kleinman (1991), anthropologist and psychiatrist, criticizes psychiatry today for showing even less interest in cultural themes with the rise in biological influence. He points out that psychiatry as a discipline has its roots firmly in western culture. Most of its key figures have been European or North American. He asks us to question whether psychiatry can be considered to be a 'science' if its knowledge base is limited to research from middle-class whites in North America, the United Kingdom and western Europe. But although the influence of psychiatry extends well beyond middle-class western culture, there is no doubt that psychiatry developed in a particular time and period in *western* society. And psychiatry, more than any other branch of medicine, has to be understood in a broad socio-political context, which must take into account ethnicity, culture and politics both inside and outside the sphere of health care. In Chapter 4, I explore the political, social and cultural pressures on a profession which has constantly sought to define and redefine its scope and the limits of its expertise.

I have little doubt that many of my fellow psychiatrists will disagree with what I have written about the profession in this book. I finally decided to study psychiatry after reading Anthony Clare's masterpiece, *Psychiatry in Dissent* (1980), and I have never regretted my decision. What makes my profession so fascinating is its complexity, which provides opportunity and room for both creativity and dissenting opinions, and I hope that my enthusiasm for my chosen career shines through. I have tried to be even-handed but honest in my discussion of different points of view, however I have no doubt that my particular prejudices will be readily apparent to the reader. My own experience of growing up in a family with a sibling who has mental illness, and my own treatment for episodes of depression during my adult life, have undoubtedly influenced my view of the world of mental health and illness. My own personal view of the future of psychiatry, with reference to the literature on this topic, can be found in Chapter 5.

Further information on psychiatry as a career can be found in Appendix 1 and terms in bold print in the main text are defined in Appendix 2.

Linda Gask

Manchester 2003

1

PSYCHIATRY: HISTORICAL CONTEXT OF A PROFESSION

There are many possible and conflicting histories of psychiatry (Newnes 1999). Histories of psychiatry may focus on treatment, disorder, institutions, professionals and, not least, patients themselves and their experiences of care and treatment by the profession. The aim of this chapter is, first, to help the reader understand the history of the ideas that have influenced psychiatric thinking today and, second, to try to set out a meaningful chronology of the development of the profession of psychiatry and its institutions. It does not aim to be a comprehensive history of psychiatry, but a presentation of relevant highlights to contextualize the development of the profession.

Before psychiatry

The medicalization of madness began in the time of the Ancient Greeks. Hippocratic medicine explained health and illness in terms of humours or 'basic juices'. The theory of Humoral Balance explained the temperaments, or what would in later centuries be called 'personality' and 'psychological dispositions'. Humoral thinking was essentially holistic and could explain both the psychological and physical without difficulty. The problem in differentiating 'mind' from 'body' would come only in the eighteenth century with the influence of Cartesian dualism on medical thinking (see Porter 2002). As it was impossible for the soul to be 'ill', mental illness was in a sense a contradiction in terms. Physical causes would be (and still are) sought for mental symptoms.

A distinction must be drawn here, however, between the progress in understanding the science of mental life and the practice of caring for the mentally ill. Humane treatment of the mentally ill was not widely practised before the late eighteenth century and in many countries is still not the norm even today. Edward Shorter in his key historic text, the most readable history of psychiatry published in the last decade, comments that:

One may abandon immediately any romantic notion of the insane in past times as being permitted to gambol on the village green or ruminate idly in the shadow of the oak tree. Before the middle of the nineteenth century, the people of villages and small towns had a horror of those who were different, an authoritarian intolerance of behaviour that did not conform to rigidly drawn norms. (Shorter 1997: 2)

People who were strange or different and not tolerated in society were cared for in their own families, often restrained, or sent to asylums, which existed from early times. In seventeenth-century England, people still resorted to advice from priests and astrologers when they had serious personal problems or worries (Thomas 1971).

It was not until the end of the eighteenth century that doctors first appeared who believed that treatment required addressing the patient's psyche rather than her body. Even Benjamin Rush, officially acknowledged by the American Psychiatric Association as the 'father of American psychiatry', believed that the best remedy was bloodletting. Changes began to occur, in part due to an uptake of new philosophical theories of sensation and perception. William Cullen, at the University of Edinburgh Medical School, coined the term *neurosis* meaning some 'inequality in the excitement of the brain'. Cullen also began to formulate the idea of mental illness as something grounded in 'dynamic neurophysiology' (Porter 2002: 128). At a more public level, Francis Willis treated the mad King George the Third of England in the late eighteenth century, utilizing a partially psychological approach by which he attempted to outwit the deluded psyche of his patient. His therapeutic style was a mixture of bullying, encouragement, and 'fixing with the eye' (Porter 2002: 103), and he did apparently achieve some therapeutic success at first. It is paradoxical that a more recent critique of the king's illness suggests that he was indeed suffering from a physical disorder which has psychological concomitants, acute intermittent porphyria (Hunter and MacAlpine 1963).

But it was the broader changes that started to occur across Europe that really began to revolutionize not only society but also the care of the mentally ill and to put down the foundations of psychiatry as we know it today.

The humane reformers

The asylum was not instituted before the practice of psychiatry; psychiatry rather was the practice developed to manage its inmates. (Porter 2002: 100)

It is impossible to write a history of psychiatry without considering the history of the institution in which so many psychiatrists, even today, have trained. Madhouses existed long before the eighteenth century. Indeed the religious priory of St Mary of Bethlem – forerunner of Bedlam, housed lunatics from 1377. However, it was in the eighteenth century that madhouses really began to multiply in numbers. Certainly, in no country was medical supervision a legal requirement before 1800 (in the UK this was 1828), nor did it automatically ensure good care. Some of the best initiatives were run by lay people such as the Retreat at York, which was run by Quakers, but a series of parliamentary Acts passed from the 1820s required medical presence first in public and later in private asylums. Asylums varied considerably in quality but almost all at that time used physical restraints such as the straitjacket, still in use today in many parts of the world.

But at the beginning of the nineteenth century progressive thinkers began to believe that if insanity was a mental disorder it required a mental treatment. This came about in the context of Enlightenment thinking, whereby physicians began to believe that through the use of reason and science they could improve on the care and treatment of previous generations. A new generation of physicians was filled not only with the confidence in their ability to heal, but also in the healing power of the asylum itself. William Battie,[1] who was the founding medical officer at St Luke's Hospital asylum in London and at one point President of the College of Physicians, promoted the asylum as a place of treatment and pronounced madness 'as manageable as many other distempers, which are equally dreadful and obstinate, and yet not looked upon as incurable' (Battie 1758: 93).

At the two large asylums in Paris, the Salpêtrière and Bicêtre hospitals, Dr Philippe Pinel, inspired by the revolutionary ideals of liberty, equality and fraternity, achieved fame for having struck the chains off the madmen at Bicêtre (though according to Shorter – 1997: 11 – it was probably his hospital manager who actually gave the order). What was clear, however, was that in the first half of the nineteenth century there were men who had medical degrees, such as William Tuke and John Connolly, who wanted to improve society *and* were proud to work in the new asylums, believing them to be places where effective and humane treatment could be provided.

William Tuke, a Quaker tea merchant in York, wanted to improve the care of those in his community who suffered from mental disorders. The York Retreat became famous for the kindness with which its inmates were treated. The (mostly lay) people who devised the therapeutic approach practised at the Retreat believed that kindness itself would help to bring a patient back from the brink of madness. A whole new approach to treatment known as *moral therapy* was developed, in effect something between counselling and what would later be called 'milieu therapy'.[2]

Across Europe and America the numbers of patients admitted to asylums increased. At the beginning of the century physicians specializing in mental disorders, such as Samuel B. Woodward at the Worcester State Hospital and Pliny Earle of the Bloomingdale asylum in New York, both in the USA, managed to provide a model of care which integrated both medical and moral therapies in a climate of therapeutic optimism. They are listed as among the thirteen originators of the Association of Medical Superintendents of American Institutions for the Insane which was established in 1844 and later became the American Psychiatric Association.

Two key pioneers in England who introduced non-restraint in the 1830s were Robert Gardiner-Hill at the Lincoln asylum and John Connolly at the New Middlesex County Lunatic Asylum at Hanwell in West London. Hill and Connolly renounced all forms of mechanical coercion whatsoever: not just irons and manacles but fabric cuffs and straitjackets too. These were replaced by surveillance by trained attendants and a 'regime of labour which would stimulate the mind and discipline the body' (Porter 2002: 114). The asylum became a self-sufficient community with its own farm laundries and workshops. Throughout the nineteenth century numbers continued to rise and safeguards against improper confinement were extended until, in the Lunacy Act of 1890, two medical certificates were now required for the detention of all patients. Psychiatrists had begun to establish themselves as experts in matters of the mind and arbiters in judging who should and should not be held responsible for their own actions, a development not viewed positively by all observers (see Hervey 1985).

The birth of the profession

The nineteenth-century word for a psychiatrist was 'alienist', which has been defined thus: 'One who was designated as an intermediary between the social world and the world of the mentally ill, he defined the relations between the two or who, in other words, was the agent of their alienation' (Littlewood and Lipsedge 1997: 33).

He (and indeed it was 'he' at this time[3]) identified the mentally ill, segregated them, and, if possible, later reintroduced them into the community. Johann Christian Reil (quoted by Shorter 1997: 17) described the qualities of a good psychiatrist: 'perspicacity, a talent for observation, intelligence, good will, persistence, patience, experience, an imposing physique, and a countenance that commands respect.' In 1808 he coined the term *Psychiaterie* which he later shortened to *Psychiatrie*. Psychiatry had been born as a medical speciality.[4]

Some have argued that a major driving force in the development of *professionalization* was psychiatrists, then known commonly as alienists, seeking to expand their wealth and power. Andrew Scull (1979) has particularly lambasted psychiatry in his writings about the asylum era. He argues that psychiatry sought to wrest control of the asylum from lay administrators in order to gain wealth and power, and underpinned this by constructing a knowledge base to justify a medical authority over lunacy. Certainly those psychiatrists who owned and operated private madhouses did make a great deal of money, both at this time and afterwards.

In 1841 the Association of Medical Officers of Asylums and Hospitals for the Insane was formed, later to become the Royal Medico Psychological Association and finally, in 1971, the Royal College of Psychiatrists. It first published the *Asylum Journal* in 1853 but renamed it the *Journal of Mental Science* in 1858. (It is now the *British Journal of Psychiatry*.) The journal was actually founded by Sir John Charles Bucknell, who with Daniel Hack Tuke published in 1858 the first major psychiatric text in English, *Psychological Medicine*. The forerunner of the American Psychiatric Association similarly began in 1844 as the Association of Medical Superintendents of American Institutions for the Insane.

In Germany there was a strong link between psychiatry and neurology, especially at the academic 'neuropsychiatric' clinics in universities, which had been promoted by the distinguished German psychiatrist Griesinger. Elsewhere across Europe and America there was much less of a link between neurology and psychiatry. Neurology, the speciality concerned with the diagnosis and treatment of nervous disorders, emerged in the middle of the nineteenth century as one of the earliest specialities to exist in medicine. Neurologists then, unlike today, were involved in treating not only physical disorders of the brain and nervous system but also other complaints that were clearly more psychological in origin. This distinction between the two specialities would have an impact on the history of the treatment of mental illness in the western world.

The first organic psychiatrists

Psychiatry has typically pursued twin goals: gaining a scientific grasp of mental illness, and healing the mentally ill. These have generally been seen as inseparable, but at times one has been emphasized more than another. Looking back to the later years of the nineteenth century it is possible to identify an important parallel with the end of the twentieth century: the growing belief that the answer to mental disorder lay in a better understanding of brain pathology. Reil himself was in no doubt as to the biological basis of madness. After him, a succession of distinguished, mostly German, neuropsychiatrists such as Alzheimer, Pick and Wernicke, now household names in neuropathology, attempted to identify a real biomedical basis for mental disturbance. But the growth in psychiatric research was simply part of the clinical-pathological movement sweeping through medicine as a whole. Most of this work took place not in asylums but in universities. At the same time, teaching in psychiatry became organized in the university departments. In all of these tasks German psychiatrists were pre-eminent. However, these organically focused doctors were undoubtedly far more interested in discovering diseases than they were in talking to their patients.

In Britain the leading psychiatrist of the era was Henry Maudsley (see Lewis 1950), who at the age of 24 was appointed medical Superintendent of the Manchester Royal Lunatic Hospital, later (and still) known as Cheadle Royal. Three years later he moved to London to take up the editorship of the *Journal of Mental Science*. It is worth noting also that Maudsley had married the youngest daughter of John Connolly, one of the great pioneers of psychiatry, who died a month after the wedding of his daughter. Maudsley had the good luck to take over the lease of his late father-in-law's clinic and thus, with his own private consulting practice, became a wealthy man. Maudsley too was convinced that 'mind disease' was 'brain disease'. In 1907 he donated money to the London County Council for a new asylum, on condition that it accept only people who had recently become ill and make provision for teaching and research. However, it was only in 1923 that the Maudsley Hospital in Denmark Hill, south London, became the facility that he had envisioned 'for exact scientific research on the causes and pathology of mental diseases'. A Chair in Psychiatry was not appointed until 1936.

But anatomy and physiology, so helpful in the broader field of medicine, failed to teach the alienist anything about the nature of the illnesses in the patients that he saw progressively filling up his wards in the asylum,[5] except in the case of syphilis where an infective agent had indeed been identified.[6] Griesinger himself came to believe that mental diseases were typically progressive, leading to chronic irreversible brain degeneration. Hereditary factors were also believed to play a part. Benedict-Augustin Morel, a Frenchman who was a physician to two large asylums, turned **degeneration** into an influential explanatory principle in his treatise on physical and moral degeneration (Morel 1857). He thought that this was produced by both organic and social factors and was cumulative over the generations. His nihilism was mirrored by an increasing therapeutic pessimism among those working in the asylums. Both the alienists and their patients were stigmatized.

Life as an asylum doctor

As a medical student in the 1890s, the future psychoanalyst Ernest Jones once heard a friend speculate about what asylum doctors or alienists discussed at their meetings: ' "I suppose," his friend said, "they read papers on an improved variety of the Chubb lock" ' (Shepherd 2002: 6). Jones's point was that alienists were in fact just glorified jailers. By 1913 there were 165,000 registered lunatics in Britain's asylums – 78,000 men and 87,000 women – and the medical press was full of complaints from alienists about the isolation and backwardness of their profession. The reputation of psychiatrists among other doctors was low. Ernest Jones also told the story of a medical superintendent of an asylum who was desperate to employ an assistant medical officer and stated that the qualifications did not matter too much provided that the doctor could play cricket with the patients (Turner 1999). Since half a dozen doctors were likely to be looking after more than 2,000 patients it seemed unlikely that any kind of therapy could be sustained. It was enough to carry out successfully routine documentation and feeding.

Life as an asylum doctor would not change considerably for another half-century.

Neurology and psychiatry

By the beginning of the twentieth century there were clearly two parallel tracks to diagnosis and treatment of mental disorder. Those people who were psychotic or otherwise severely mentally ill were cared for in asylums by alienists, or to a more limited degree as outpatients by neurologists. However, those people with less severe disorders for which no physical cause could be found and who mostly received the diagnoses of **hysteria** and neurasthenia were, if they could afford to pay, treated privately by neurologists. These disorders were considered to be on the increase. An American neurologist, George Beard, coined the term *neurasthenia*, which he considered was a disease of civilization 'brought about by the complex agencies of modern life'.[7] The stock treatment for neurasthenia was the cure devised by the Philadelphia neurologist Silas Weir Mitchell, which involved isolation, entire bed-rest and excessive feeding with a milk diet. Successful, powerful and wealthy neurologists such as Mitchell looked down scornfully at psychiatrists and their treatment: 'Whatever the gullible public might believe about your therapy we [neurologists] hold the reverse opinion and think your hospitals are never to be used save as the last resource' (Weir Mitchell quoted in Shorter 1997: 68).

Patients, then as now perhaps, undoubtedly found the idea of suffering from a physical disorder of the nerves far less worrying and potentially stigmatizing than suffering from a mental illness. However, increasingly sophisticated investigation of the nervous system failed to produce any confirmation of the hypothesis that the neurasthenia was due to depletion of the body's nerve force. Despite removal from neurology textbooks the diagnosis has survived to the present day for reasons to do with its very vagueness. It managed (and still manages) to explain subjective bodily symptoms in terms of objective physical disease, thus removing any suggestion of the patient's own culpability in them.

The 'nervous breakdown' became the disease of the Edwardian age. Many famous literary figures were treated privately by eminent neurologists, not least Virginia Woolf, who did indeed suffer from a major psychiatric illness: **bipolar disorder**. More commonly, however, it was the wealthy neurotic patient suffering from 'nerves' who saw the neurologist privately, while ordinary working people tried an increasing number of patent remedies advertised in the developing media. When a wealthy person with a psychotic illness required hospitalization they would be admitted to one of the private asylums where conditions were somewhat better than in the grossly over-crowded county hospitals. Class distinctions would persist and grow further with the arrival of psychoanalysis.

The beginnings of modern psychiatry

Emil Kraepelin was born at about the same time as Sigmund Freud. His father was an actor, opera singer and music teacher who even-tually became a travelling storyteller with something of a drink problem (see Engstrom and Weber 1999). Emil was raised by his mother but carried a strong conviction of the degenerative influence of alcohol throughout his life. His great contribution to psychiatry was that he began to explore the longitudinal development of his patients' illnesses, believing that by examining the entire course of an illness he could uncover the unique characteristics of natural disease entities. He used an ingenious card-filing system to collect, sort and compare clinical information on his patients and specifically observed and documented patients' illnesses over extended periods of time. By these methods he was able to describe the two major disease entities that we recognize today, which he called **dementia praecox** and **manic-depressive psychosis**. Kraepelin was not a biological psychiatrist but there is no doubt that being a 'Kraepelinian' psychiatrist meant that one operated within a medical model rather than a biopsychosocial model.

The legacy of Kraepelin remains with us today in both of the major classification systems in use in the world – the *Diagnostic and Statistical Manual* (*DSM* – used by the Americans and worldwide) and the *International Classification of Disease* (*ICD* – used throughout the world but not in America). It is evident that Kraepelin and his work was rediscovered by American psychiatry in the last quarter of the twentieth century when psychiatry shifted back towards tighter diagnosis and classification (see page 28). Kraepelin put considerable emphasis on the importance of the course of the illness in arriving at a diagnosis, and also pioneered psychological testing for psychiatric patients. What his neuropathological colleagues, Alzheimer and Nissl, were able to explain on the basis of neuroanatomical abnormality, they finally declared to be the remit of neurology. But it was Kraepelin who, in carving out the field of emotional disorder that was to be the remit of psychiatrists, shaped modern psychiatry.

Adolf Meyer was a contemporary of Kraepelin who took things in quite a different direction. Meyer qualified in medicine in Switzerland and studied in France and Britain before taking up the opportunity of a career in America where he eventually became established at Johns Hopkins University. He used the term 'psychobiology' to indicate a method of looking at the whole person and considered a wide range of factors in the aetiology of mental illness. Most radically he did not attempt to solve the mind–body conflict but put great store on seeing the patient as a product of his psychological, social and biological heritage. A detailed assessment of the patient's life experience, known as a life chart, would be drawn up. Meyer was particularly influential in British psychiatry through the teaching of Aubrey Lewis (see Gelder 1991). Meyer respected the value of Kraepelin's diagnostic system but warned against what he considered the potential misuse of simplistic diagnostic categories.

Although Kraepelin described **dementia praecox**, which we now know as **schizophrenia**, he did not coin the term. Credit for this must go to Eugen Bleuler, a Swiss psychiatrist who was Professor of Psychiatry in Zürich until 1927. Bleuler's primary symptom of schizophrenia was cognitive in form: a type of thought disorder with **loosening of associations**. Bleuler provides the link between more orthodox psychiatry and the theories of the unconscious devised by the psychoanalysts. His views led to more therapeutic optimism, but at the same time his looser approach to diagnosis unfortunately led psychiatrists in the USA to label people with few or no symptoms as having schizophrenia. In the USSR, some psychiatrists used the extraordinary diagnosis of 'sluggish schizophrenia' for people who dissented politically (see Chapter 4).

The German pre-eminence in the field of psychopathology continued well into the 20th century. Indeed Germany led the field of psychiatric research until the arrival of the Nazis and the Third Reich in 1933. Karl Jaspers, a psychiatrist and philosopher, produced his book *General Psychopathology* (1913), which also had a considerable influence on the training of psychiatrists in the UK. Jaspers is of particular importance in the history of psychiatry because he brings together in his work the rigour of classification, an emphasis on empathic understanding and an understanding of phenomenology. But in 1937 Jaspers was forbidden to teach or publish any longer. What was his crime? His wife was Jewish.

The psychoanalysts

Towards the end of the nineteenth century, partly in reaction to the pessimism of asylum psychiatry and the dogmatism of the organic psychiatrists, a new style of psychiatry that we can recognize now as *dynamic* began to appear. Dynamic psychiatry was not conceived by Sigmund Freud but by Pierre Janet at the Salpêtrière in Paris. He spent considerable time researching **hysteria** and the neuroses but has been a largely forgotten figure in the history of psychiatry, much overshadowed by Freud himself. Janet, like Freud, was a neurologist, albeit a very psychologically minded one. He followed Jean-Marie Charcot who had been a professor of neurology and one of the first doctors to take hysteria seriously, successfully using hypnosis as a treatment. He showed that by experimenting with hypnosis, hysterical symptoms such as paralysis of the arm could be artificially produced and then removed. Janet produced comprehensive clinical descriptions of **hysteria, anorexia, amnesia,** and **obsessional neuroses** – and of their treatment with hypnosis, suggestion and other psychodynamic techniques (see Brown 1999).

It is difficult to achieve the right balance with respect to psychoanalysis and other branches of the history of psychiatry. If this book had been written even thirty years ago the size of the section devoted to Freud and his followers would probably have been much larger. The influence of psychoanalysis on psychiatry as it is practised in the United States has been immense and was always much greater than in Europe – a fact which surprises young psychiatrists today, who see America as the home of biological psychiatry *par excellence*. This is not the place to explore in any detail the conceptual issues at the base of psychoanalysis but instead I would like to try and demonstrate how the psychoanalytic movement has influenced the way in which psychiatrists work today. We shall return to this theme again in the second chapter of this book. Psychoanalysis itself originated in the late 1890s through informal exchanges between a small group of psychiatrists, neurologists, writers, lawyers and sociologists in France, Germany and central Europe. Freud, an Austrian neurologist, entered into extensive correspondence with colleagues such as Josef Breuer and Wilhelm Fliess, and coined the term *psychoanalysis* in 1896.

At an early stage Freud began to believe that sexual abuse of children directly contributed to the development of mental disorder in later life. This has subsequently become known as his 'seduction theory'. Later he refined and qualified his view, suggesting that fantasy rather than reality was playing a key part. This has led some later writers, such as Masson (1992), to accuse Freud of backtracking from the truth.

Freud intended the term 'psychoanalysis' to apply both to the technique of working with mental disorders and to an interpretive method that could be applied widely in both social and human sciences. Freud confessed that he had 'never been a therapeutic enthusiast' (Stanton 1999: 41) and both of his early innovatory books, *The Interpretation of Dreams* (1900) and *The Psychopathology of Everyday Life* (1901), were really intended to address the specific form and function of the unconscious process rather than be seen as expositions of clinical experience. Clinical psychoanalysis at first rarely lasted more than a few months. But later treatments lasted much longer, prompted apparently by work with psychotic and borderline patients (something that Freud apparently advised against but which became common practice in US psychiatry in the middle part of the twentieth century).

By the time of the first International Psychoanalytic Association meeting in Nuremberg in 1910 splits were beginning to appear in the psychoanalytic movement. Two Viennese medical psychoanalysts,

Alfred Adler and Wilhelm Stekel, expressed their opposition to the nomination of Carl Gustav Jung as president. Both of them went on to develop their own approaches to therapy. Later, a split occurred too between Freud and Jung, who went on to develop his own school of 'analytic psychology'. Many others, too numerous to mention here, were also influential in the development of psychoanalysis throughout Europe. Of particular note are Melanie Klein who came from Berlin to the United Kingdom, Anna Freud who founded the practice of child psychoanalysis, Karen Horney and Wilhelm Reich. By the end of the second decade of the twentieth century psychoanalysis had grown from its early informal structure into an international institution with national societies, affiliated groups and a formalized training structure for analysts, including the requirement that all trainees should undergo personal analysis themselves. The issue of whether all applicants needed to be medically qualified was controversial. Most American analysts argued they should (later in the century all American psychiatrists would receive analytic training, unlike in Europe where this was much less common) but the Europeans, following Freud, saw an important role for non-medical analysts. At this time psychoanalysts also began to infiltrate universities. From the time of the Great War onwards psychoanalysis began to have a significant impact on the way that psychiatry was practised. The treatment of neurosis was no longer left to neurologists but began to be taken up by psychiatrists, keen to leave the asylum for a least part of the week to see patients in their private consulting rooms.

Psychoanalysis established itself not only as a medical treatment but as a major cultural force in the twentieth century. In the future when lay people thought about psychiatrists they were as likely to imagine the analyst's couch as the asylum ward. Yet that was in fact not the reality for the majority of people in the world who sought mental health care, but rather for a privileged few who were treated privately.

Psychiatrists in war

The impact of the Great War and later conflicts on the developments in psychiatry during the twentieth century continues to be debated. Much has been written about *shell-shock*, a term first used by British soldiers in 1914 and taken up by medicine and the army soon afterwards. The experience of war had a considerable impact on how psychiatrists perceived the nature of mental disorder and how they proposed to treat it. As Ben Shepherd, the historian, has observed:

Psychiatrists saw the effects of battle on the human mind and recorded them with wonderful eloquence. War horrified, appalled, yet also excited them. It provided an extreme environment, a laboratory in which every theory could be tested literally to destruction; war shattered the mind, but in an intellectually absorbing way. (Shepherd 2002: xvii)

Shepherd (1999) has described four phases in the debate that took place about how to treat shell-shock. During the first phase, which he calls 'initial bewilderment', the authorities and doctors were quite overwhelmed by what they saw and simply did not know how to respond. Many soldiers showed peculiar physical and psychological symptoms about which there was considerable debate. The great French neurologist Joseph Babinski considered these to be physically caused. However, it gradually became clear, during the second phase that the majority of these cases were indistinguishable from the neurotic disorders seen in the general population. Skilled therapists could achieve a rapid cure. However, many began to use what would now be considered quite brutal physical treatments including Faradism, which involved applying an electric current to the affected body part. Once again, class distinctions began to appear with the utilization, in the third phase, of psychoanalysis, but only for officers. Pat Barker's novel *Regeneration* (1992) skilfully brings to life the meeting between the poet Siegfried Sassoon and the psychologist, W.H. Rivers at Craiglockhart Hospital, Edinburgh. W.H. Rivers' extraordinary career, which spanned physiology, anthropology and psychology, is summarized in Bewley (1998). In the last phase, there was finally an attempt to marry together psychological and physical factors in a way that foreshadowed modern psychosomatic theories.

The psychiatrists who went to the front were not necessarily welcomed by the men they were there to treat. Nicknames such as 'trick cyclist' and 'shrink' were invented for them. But the war was to change psychiatry, and the way that it was viewed by society. Able men, of previously 'good character' had been shown to go 'mad' under conditions of war. Mental illness seemed to become less 'alien' and a newer type of doctor, one who no longer wanted to be an 'alienist', would eventually emerge to discover, describe and treat 'common mental health problems'.[8]

Pioneers of physical treatment

During the first half of the twentieth century the number of patients admitted to mental hospitals, as the asylums now began to be called, continued to rise. At the same time, the rate of recovery dropped from 40 per cent in the 1870s to 31 per cent in the 1920s, and it began to be asked whether scientific psychiatry had failed. David Clark, who later became a pioneer of social psychiatry, described the typical asylum scene in the first half of the twentieth century:

> You were taken in by somebody with a key, who unlocked the door and then locked it behind you. The crashing of the keys in the locks was an essential part of asylum life then, just as it is today in jails. You'd be shown into a big bare room, overcrowded with people, with scrubbed floors, bare wooden tables, benches screwed in the floors. People milling around in shapeless clothing. There was a smell in the air of urine, paraldehyde, floor polish, boiled cabbage, and carbolic soap – the asylum smell. (Clark 1985: 78)

We generally think of the second half of the twentieth century as the time when major steps were made in developing treatments in psychiatry, but the early work was carried out by pioneers, some now forgotten, in the twenties and thirties in response to the urgent need to try and find effective treatments. Julius Wagner-Jauregg, the only psychiatrist ever to have been awarded the Nobel Prize (in 1927), studied and practised in Vienna. His 'fever cure' produced by infecting patients suffering from neurosyphilis with malaria did not survive as a treatment following the introduction of penicillin. However, it was a major step forward in looking for physical treatments for the psychoses, and there are psychiatrists alive today who can still remember malarial mosquitoes being kept in the hospital to treat general paresis of the insane (known as GPI).

Drug treatments had been used in psychiatry from the nineteenth century with the gradual introduction of substances such as chloral and bromine. At the beginning of the twentieth century the **barbiturates** appeared, and were used both in hospitals and in the community. Their ability to induce prolonged deep sleep led to the development of deep sleep therapy by Jakob Klaesi in Switzerland. Deep sleep therapy became widely adopted for severe psychotic mood disorders. By the end of the 1920s the discipline of **psychopharmacology** was becoming established in psychiatry.

The 1930s, however, saw far more dramatic steps forward in physical treatments, the ramifications of which are still felt today. Three events occurred at about the same time – the development of **electro-convulsive therapy (ECT)**, **insulin coma treatment** and **psychosurgery**. Manfred Sakel was developing his insulin coma treatment in Vienna during the same period that Ladislaus von Meduna, a researcher in Budapest who was exploring the comparative neuropathology of dementia praecox and epilepsy, developed the method of inducing seizures with a substance called

Metrazol as a form of treatment for **dementia praecox**. Further research indicated that it was the seizure rather than the specific substance given to induce it that was effective.

In an experiment that would never today get through the preliminary stages of an ethical committee, Ugo Cerletti and Luigi Bini, working in Rome, famously induced a grand mal seizure by means of an electric current in a 39-year-old man suffering from a psychotic episode. He had been admitted to the University Hospital, having been found wandering about in the railway station. After eleven applications of what Cerletti called *electro-shock treatment* the patient fortunately made a complete recovery, but the same could not be said for many other patients who received poorly tested, risky and unsound therapies during this period. Tens of thousands of people on both sides of the Atlantic were given a **leucotomy**, a procedure pioneered by Antonio Caetanode Abreu Freire Egas Moniz (1927), a Portuguese neurologist who was also awarded the Nobel Prize. This period has been called by one eminent American psychiatrist 'a sad chapter in our history' (Romano 1994).

Later, ECT would only be given to patients who were fully anaesthetized and paralysed in order to prevent them injuring themselves during a fit. However, the incident in which the character played by Jack Nicholson in the film *One Flew over the Cuckoo's Nest* was given ECT has been etched on the public consciousness. ECT was attacked in the US by the psychoanalytic lobby and across the world by the anti-psychiatry lobby (see below). All of these physical treatments, including ECT, are today viewed by the general public with considerable distaste, but at the time they were developed they provided real hope for effective treatment in the face of therapeutic despair (Valenstein 1986). ECT is still regularly in use – if less than in the recent past, but insulin coma treatment fell out of use in the 1950s following the arrival of chlorpromazine. Psychosurgery is still performed today in a small number of centres utilizing very precise lesions in the brain, and although selection criteria are very clearly defined, with a focus on intractable depression and anxiety, it remains controversial.

Nazi psychiatry

When the remains of the last two of almost 800 children and babies who died in Vienna in the 1930s were finally laid to rest in April 2002 (Connolly 2002), few people living now would perhaps understand the significance of this event. All becomes clear when one learns that these children were killed during the Nazi regime's euthanasia programme, a fact made no less unpalatable by the knowledge that certain Viennese scientists were still arguing that a further 1,000 brain specimens, which might have come from other child victims, were too valuable as scientific specimens to hand over. Collection of the specimens had been partly presided over by Dr Heinrich Gross who had been head of the Spiegelgrund clinic in Vienna for two years during the Second World War. He was remembered by a survivor of the clinic, who at the time had been a 10-year-old boy with a diagnosis of syphilis, as a quiet and hardworking man who always wore his brown Nazi uniform on the wards. He also recalled that some of his friends were taken away and he never saw them again. What happened to German psychiatry and psychiatrists during the Nazi regime of the 1930s?

During the Germany of the 1920s psychoanalysis had been developing rapidly and there had been particularly important developments in child psychotherapy. But after Hitler became Chancellor in 1933, eugenics and 'social Darwinism' philosophies that had been around since the end of the nineteenth century, began to become influential in a particularly ominous way. The killing of children began after a family asked Hitler for permission to have their handicapped child killed. Hitler instructed his personal physician Karl Brandt to kill not only that child, but others who were similarly disabled. The killings escalated and more than 5,000 children, including those who were labelled as delinquents, were killed. Undoubtedly several psychiatrists were involved. Many children died from an overdose of drugs, but others, apparently, died during 'research' activities.

At the same time many other psychiatrists were attempting to leave Germany. Those who were Jewish were particularly at risk, but Jewish psychoanalysts, who practised treatment developed by Freud, a Jew, were doubly so. Sigmund Freud himself emigrated to Britain, where he died in 1939. However, the majority of German and Austrian psychiatrists and psychoanalysts who fled from the Nazis went to America. This was to have a major impact on developments in American psychiatry and the direction that it would take for the next forty years.

In Germany, Nazi psychiatry began to develop its own theory and practice, which owed something to the legacy of Kraepelin who had latterly written extensively about degeneration theories and the need for protection of the populace from disorders such as alcoholism, syphilis and homosexuality, ultimately by biological engineering. In 1933, the Nazis launched a 'Law for the Prevention of Offspring with Hereditary Diseases'. All German doctors were required to read the Swiss psychiatrist Ernst Rudin's book, which proposed extinction of patients with the diagnoses of dementia and alcoholism. Many departments of psychiatry were implicated in the Holocaust that followed, in which 300,000 psychiatric patients were put to death. Of particular note must be the Munich psychiatric institute of which Kurt Schneider had been director since 1931 and the department in Würzburg where Professor Heyde became a member of the SAS and the psychiatric expert for the Gestapo (Peters 1999). Psychotherapy survived the Nazi purge, but the Nazis declared that a new Psychotherapeutic Association should be founded, and its new president, a cousin of Hermann Goering, declared that Hitler's *Mein Kampf* should be the basic text.

In the midst of all of this there were episodes of great courage and resistance. Hans Gerhard Creutzfeldt, who had described Creutzfeldt–Jakob disease, dared to criticize the Nazis in his lectures and was interrogated on a number of occasions. Many psychiatrists refused to participate – at the expense of their careers. But the name of Bonhoeffer is less remembered for the work of the father, Karl, Professor of Psychiatry in Berlin, who described acute organic syndromes of the brain, than for the bravery of his sons, one of whom, Dietrich (the theologist) became an important symbol to those who dared to resist Hitler. Dietrich and his brother Klaus were both hanged in a concentration camp in 1945.

When the World Psychiatric Association held its congress in Hamburg in 1999 the death of so many people at the hands of those who purported to care for them was remembered both in a moving exhibition and by demonstrations by mental health workers and patients who felt that it was still too soon for such a meeting to come to Germany. The most moving exhibits were the letters from relatives inquiring about their loved ones who had disappeared (Madden 2000).

We will explore more recent interactions between psychiatry and political ideology (in Soviet Russia and China) in Chapter 4.

The Second World War and the origins of social psychiatry

It was an émigré Jewish physician and psychotherapist, Joshua Bierer, who began to organize psychotherapy groups, first for inpatients at Runwell Hospital in Essex in the late-1930s and later for outpatients at two London teaching hospitals, Guy's and St Bartholomew's. Meanwhile, changes in the law in Britain had begun to lay the ground for greater accessibility of treatment with the passing of the Mental Treatment Act of 1930, which stipulated that there should be no distinction between mental and physical treatments. Treatment should be available to everyone who wanted it, without certification, voluntarily wherever and whenever possible.

By the time of the Second World War pychotherapeutic treatments had begun to prove their value in managing men who were evacuated from the front line with psychological problems, and in getting them successfully back to work again. The psychoanalytic influence on army psychiatry was inevitable given the role of J.R. Rees, who had co-founded the Tavistock Clinic in London, an outpatient unit which offered psychoanalytically informed treatment to patients with neurotic illnesses. In 1939, Rees took up the post of director of army psychiatry, bringing with him a group of young and enthusiastic psychoanalytically orientated psychiatrists including Tom Main and John Bowlby, later to be famous for his work on attachment theory. Psychoanalytically trained psychiatrists also influenced the process of officer selection.

At Northfield Military Hospital in Birmingham several key figures came together for the first time, including the psychoanalyst Wilfred Bion, S.H. Foulkes, another refugee from Europe who later developed the technique of group analysis, and the psychiatrist Tom Main. Here they founded the concept of the therapeutic community which they described as:

> An attempt to use a hospital not as an organisation run by doctors in the interests of their own technical efficiency, but as a community with the aim of full participation of all its members in its daily life and the central aim of resocialisation of the neurotic individual for life in organised society. (Main 1946: 66)

This change in the balance of power between staff and patients led to a freer and more self-directed approach to treatment. However, although psychoanalytic principles played a large part in the treatment provided at Northfield, barbiturate narcosis and ECT were also used.

At the same time, another key figure in the foundation of social psychiatry, Maxwell Jones, was working at Mill Hill School in North London, to which the Maudsley Hospital had been evacuated during the war. In his approach to therapy, Maxwell Jones rejected psychoanalysis in favour of ideas drawn broadly from social psychology: 'Our aim was to create an environment conducive to social maturation. It had a "family" atmosphere – no locked doors, no drugs, first names only (staff and patients) and an essentially democratic social structure' (Jones 1983: 55).

At Mill Hill some of the earliest experiments with small and large group therapy were tried out on service personnel. Later, the Mill

Hill group was asked to take over a unit in Dartford, Kent, for the treatment of returning prisoners-of-war with *combat fatigue*. Maxwell Jones went on to found what would later become the Henderson Hospital, probably the most famous therapeutic community in the world. Tom Main similarly went on to run the Cassel hospital. After the war, Bierer set up what was the first psychiatric day hospital in Britain in two war-damaged houses in Hampstead.

The concept of social psychiatry brings together a number of different ideas: the open asylum, from which patients might come and go at will; the existence of community resources which can provide care; the outpatient clinic (such clinics began to appear in European hospitals in the 1920s). Social psychiatrists saw the cause of patients' problems as neither in their biology nor in their early childhood but in their environment. The British interest in this field resonated with the political changes taking place in the Britain of the late 1940s where there was a widespread belief that the community had a responsibility to its members and where a National Health Service (NHS) was developing. The main buildings inheritance of the NHS was a system in Britain of over 100 asylums with an average population of over 1,000 patients each.

David Clark surprised his colleagues by taking the post of medical superintendent of Fulbourn Hospital in Cambridge after serving in northern Europe and the Far East as a parachute regiment medical officer. He wanted to improve the conditions of long-stay patients at the hospital and was fascinated by the social approaches that had been developed. The experience of war and its aftermath seemed to have been important:

> It was these experiences that taught me of the extraordinary things that men did to one another and the immense effect that the environment had on people. I developed a clear view of the power of social factors to help people to change. (Clark 1985: 74)

He went on to apply the principles of the therapeutic community approach to the general psychiatric hospital, attempting to undo the damage done by institutional abuse, and bringing to hospital care a psychologically informed administration.

Life in the asylums at that time had changed very little although there had been some developments with the coming of the National Health Service in 1948. All senior asylum doctors became consultants, but no one really wanted to be a superintendent because it was not considered to be a high-status job and carried a considerable administrative burden. The wards were still full of chronically ill patients. For the junior doctor there were no clinical meetings, no journal clubs and no adequate library facilities, but the food was considered to be good as asylums had their own farms. Post-war rationing went unnoticed, with a good supply of free milk, cream and vegetables. But the everyday routine for the doctor was somewhat limited. A junior doctor would have some chronic wards to look after where his job was to prescribe sedatives and make the periodic physical and mental examinations of the patients as legally required by the Board of Control. Looking back at these notes now we see that they are often a very limited record, with frequently just the words 'no change' written every year for decades. The twentieth century was late to reach the asylum.

But a revolution in health care was taking place. In Britain, in the context of the NHS, the need for a formal training in psychiatry was recognized and medical schools began to improve the teaching of psychiatry with the appointment of several new Chairs in psychiatry across the UK.[9] Outpatient clinics, day hospitals and hostels began to appear. New therapists were engaged to provide education, occupational therapy, music, art and physical activities. Doors were unlocked, allowing more freedom to patients and enabling graduated discharge. Meanwhile in London, at the Institute of Psychiatry, Aubrey Lewis built a research and teaching environment that would spawn many of the influential psychiatrists of the UK and beyond in the second half of the twentieth century. In America, the National Institute of Mental Health was founded and began to encourage individual states to look at developing alternatives to hospital care. Mental health and illness were seen as being part of a broader biomedical science and the NIMH became a powerful funder of research. But a major split was occurring in US psychiatry, with psychoanalytic treatment the prevailing wisdom in private practice in the community and physical treatments much more commonly utilized in mental hospitals.

The psychopharmacologists

The 1950s saw another revolution (Healy 1997), namely the discovery of specific psychotropic medication that seemed for the first time to tackle the symptoms of mental illness rather than simply sedate the patient. However, many of these drugs, as is often the case, were discovered fortuitously to have psychotropic effects. Imipramine, for example, was simply one of a series of compounds. Originally a possible anti-histamine, it emerged that it possessed a potent anti-depressant action, but it was a decade before it was finally marketed in 1958. A number of different researchers in both the US and Europe were working on similar projects at the same time, so it is difficult to be sure exactly who was the first to discover anti-depressants, but it does seem likely that Max Lurie, an American psychiatrist, was the first to use the term 'anti-depressant' some time around 1953. Chlorpromazine was being used to treat surgical shock when Jean Delay, Professor at the psychiatric clinic of St Anne Hospital in Paris, and his assistant Pierre Deniker began to experiment with the drug as a potential anti-psychotic. Later they would coined the term **'neuroleptic'**, a term also applied to haloperidol which was developed in 1958.

The anti-depressant action of the mono-amine oxidase inhibitors was discovered during the search for a treatment for tuberculosis. Many different compounds were synthesized from the large quantity of hydralazine left over from the Nazi rocket programme of the Second World War and tested for possible actions. **Mono-Amine Oxidase Inhibitors (or MAOIs)** were widely used in the treatment of depression, particularly in treatment-resistant illness, but their use has declined in the last twenty years because of major problems of interaction with other drugs and certain foods. Chlordiazepoxide, the first of the benzodiazepines, appeared in 1955, and diazepam in 1959. By the end of the 1960s diazepam or valium was the most widely prescribed psychotropic drug in the world, not just by psychiatrists but by general practitioners, who were beginning to play a major role in the care of mental health problems.

Within a short period of time, drugs were available for treating two major conditions, **schizophrenia** and **affective disorders**. Insulin coma treatment would become defunct. ECT, however, continued to have a place in the management of major mental disorders, particularly in severe depression.

Community psychiatry

By the early 1960s major changes were occurring in psychiatry across the world. The asylum was beginning to disappear. There are a number of reasons why this started to happen but there was little in the way of policy development or planning. The social psychiatry revolution, initiated even before the Second World War when psychiatrists had first experimented with unlocking the doors of hospitals, swept in on a wave of optimism about what could be achieved with humane care, rehabilitation, the new medications and a range of community resources. Since that period the word 'community' has been widely used without any firm agreements in psychiatry about what it actually means (see Chapter 4). The first community psychiatrists aspired to set up comprehensive public services for people with mental health problems in a defined population, using the hospital itself as only one of the resources in the community. Thus, in the Salford of the 1960s Hugh Freeman attempted to set up a system of care that was integrated into the community. This incorporated a system of screening before admission (so that people did not simply arrive on the psychiatric ward), beds in the general hospital, a day-hospital service, and a range of services integrated with those provided by social services. Hugh Freeman had no illusions that his attempts at reforming services would attract extra funding but he nevertheless had considerable freedom.

When I interviewed him in 2002, Hugh Freeman told me, 'we were desperately poor in today's terms – but consultants were incredibly autonomous. As long as you didn't spend a lot of money you could do more or less what you wanted – if you had an idea you could pursue it.'

Relationships began to be built up with general practitioners who, it was increasingly recognized, provided first-line care for people with major mental health problems and the majority of care for those suffering from milder disorders. Developments such as this were clearly in line with the 1959 Mental Health Act which removed any obstacles to caring for people with serious mental health problems in the community and also, significantly, made physicians and not magistrates the final arbiters of whether a person could be detained under mental health law.

Across the UK similar services were set up, with psychiatric beds provided for the first time in general hospitals rather than in the more remote mental hospital sites. As services outside hospital began to develop, and the more enthusiastic and talented staff followed patients, the situation inside hospitals began to deteriorate, and there was a series of scandals[10] and exposés in the media. But this did not stop the general decline in the environment for both patients and staff still working in the old asylums, although many preferred the space and sense of isolation to the increasingly fraught atmosphere of the general psychiatric ward in the district general hospital. Across Europe, mental-hospital-bed occupancy dropped by a half although Italy proved to be the most radical when in 1978 under Law 180, championed by the radical psychiatrist Franco Basaglia, it passed a law making further admission of people to mental hospital illegal.

In the United States only one-fifth of patients remained in mental hospitals by the mid-1980s. But community psychiatry in the US took on a different meaning with an emphasis on a public health model of community mental health and the prevention of mental illness. This would inevitably lead to the development of services which were focused not on severe mental illness but on emotional distress and the commoner problems faced by people in disadvantaged communities. Thus, following an initiative by President Kennedy, Community Mental Health Centers (CMHCs) had been set up with the aim of providing crisis and preventative services to the community. These centres, however, failed to effectively engage people with severe and enduring mental illness and did not succeed in providing the necessary care for people with serious mental health problems living in the community – those who might once have been in the asylum. This conflict between engaging the severely mentally ill and meeting the need of the wider population experiencing anxiety and depression related to problems in everyday living, would be played out across Europe as professionals interpreted the concept of 'community care' in different ways.

However, there were other pressures that led to the move out of hospital. The availability of specific psychoactive drugs itself brought about a revolution in the management of mental health problems with the possibility of treating many more people outside a secure hospital environment. Health service costs had also been rising steeply since the end of the war and governments were keen to reduce expenditure and look for alternatives to mental hospital treatment rather than spend large amounts of money renovating nineteenth-century buildings. It was probably this reasoning, along with the very optimistic prediction of a fall in requirements for in-patient beds (Tooth and Brooke 1961) that led a Tory minister of health, Enoch Powell, to sound the death-knell of the asylum.[11] A National Hospital Plan in Britain in 1962 ruled out any more new or enlarged mental hospitals, and further developments were to occur only in district general hospitals. But change was already afoot. Policy was following the developing trends away from hospital admission as much as it was leading it (Jones 1993). And changing social attitudes towards psychiatry and mental illness would also play a part.

Anti-psychiatry

A number of different writers from a variety of disciplines attacked psychiatry with considerable force during the 1960s (Tantam 1991). Some of these came from within psychiatry itself, the most famous – indeed the very first celebrity psychiatrist – being R.D. Laing, who trained in Scotland before moving to London.[12] His *The Divided Self* (Laing 1960) became a bestseller. In it he put forward for the first time his arguments for the development of 'madness' as a reaction to living in intolerable circumstances, often seen by him as present in the person's own family. In the USA Gregory Bateson had proposed that double-bind communication in the family might be a cause of schizophrenia, and other workers had begun to pose the possibility of the **schizophrenogenic family**. This view of the cause of 'schizophrenia' was powerfully dramatized in the film *Family Life*.

Meanwhile, a broader view of psychiatric treatment in hospitals as essentially evil was given support by the writings of Michel Foucault (1965) and Erving Goffman (1961). According to Foucault, who reconsidered the history of psychiatry in *Madness and Civilization*:

> What we call psychiatric practice is a certain moral tactic contemporary with the end of the eighteenth century, preserved in the rites of asylum life, and overlaid by the myths of positivism. (Foucault 1965: 276)

Psychiatrists were coming to be viewed as agents of social control. Such a view, alien as it may seem to the well-meaning professional, is not necessarily at odds with the day-to-day motive of the psychiatrist attempting consciously to do the best for an individual patient. As Carl May, Professor of Medical Sociology at the University of Newcastle, said to me:

> It's possible for both of these motives to exist in the same time-space; it's possible for you as the psychiatrist to be exercising your professional skills in what you see as the best interests of the patient and to be doing things that they really don't like, and at the same time be an instrument of state policy, or an instrument of some grand scientific meta-narrative or some other kind of discourse. (Interviewed by the author 2003)

During the sixties, Foucault's writings had a considerable influence on anti-psychiatry. Compulsory hospitalization was condemned, and physical treatments including drugs and ECT were attacked, notably in such books and films as *One Flew over the Cuckoo's Nest*. Alternative therapies and talking treatments were promoted. R.D. Laing founded a therapeutic community at Kingsley Hall in London[13] where the best known patient to be treated was Mary Barnes, who later wrote the story of her life there (Barnes and Berke 1991). Although this unit closed, its work continues to the present through the Philadelphia Association and the Arbours Association.

Most of the psychiatrists and their mental health colleagues who embraced anti-psychiatry were avowedly left-wing in their views.

However, anti-psychiatry also had a strong libertarian 'right' wing (Sedgwick 1982). Thomas Szasz argued in *The Myth of Mental Illness* (1974) that mental illness was not illness unless clear disease could be demonstrated. If the person wished to seek help with their life problems they could do so, but they would have to pay. Szasz was himself a psychiatrist in private practice and considered state services to be agents of social control. Approaches taken by 'paternalistic' social and community psychiatrists actively to seek out people with mental illness in the community and care for them were an anathema to him. Szasz's views can now perhaps be seen to be perfectly in tune with Thatcherite and Conservative views of a health system in which the vulnerable poor are given the 'freedom of choice' to pay for their own care.

The anti-psychiatrists had a lasting impact on psychiatrists, on other mental health professionals and on patients. Anti-psychiatry undoubtedly led to much greater sensitivity to the rights of the patient and influenced psychiatry to examine its own values. But the downside was first the impact on relationships between psychiatrists and other mental health professionals, with whom conflict was ready to erupt, and second the feeling among many relatives that they were being blamed for the genesis of mental illness. We will return to exploring recent developments in this field and the growth of the user movement in the last two decades in Chapter 3.

Rediscovering Kraepelin: the classification of psychiatry

In the first half of the twentieth century European and American psychiatry diverged considerably. America had been greatly influenced by Freud and also by Adolf Meyer (see page 12) at Johns Hopkins University in Baltimore. Both of these, although very different in many ways, stressed that events in the life of the patient were the most important causes of mental illness. Both were also influential in Europe as the tide turned, for a period at least, towards social and psychological theories. But this was never as complete as it was in the US where psychoanalytic theories and approaches to treatment were supremely powerful. At the same time, it was clear that approaches to the diagnosis of mental illness differed widely on each side of the Atlantic. In 1969 researchers in London and New York (Kendell et al. 1971) compared the diagnostic habits of psychiatrists in their two countries by showing videotapes of patients to audiences of American and British psychiatrists in turn. It became clear that it was easier to obtain a diagnosis of schizophrenia in the US and that there was no systematic approach to diagnosis across the world of psychiatry. This was followed by controversy in the US over the disease status of homosexuality (which was classified as a disease in the American official manual of diagnosis in mental health, the *Diagnostic and Statistical Manual of the American Psychiatric Association (DSM) II)*, and finally by the famous Rosenhan study. Some nineteen normal subjects presented themselves to psychiatric hospitals each saying that he or she heard the word 'thud'. All were *hospitalized* and acted normally while in hospital. Yet all received a diagnosis of 'schizophrenia in remission' (Rosenhan 1973).

During the 1970s considerable changes began to occur (Wilson 1993). A group of American research psychiatrists led by Robert Spitzer developed the vastly revised *DSM–III*, which has been followed up by two further versions and is now used worldwide (the current version is *DSM–V*). This continues to compete with the WHO *International Classification of Disease (ICD)* which is now much closer to *DSM* than was previously the case. To European psychiatrists it became clear that the US had rediscovered much of the work of the great European psychopathologists of the first half of the twentieth century. To some US observers, the developments were the achievement of a '*neo-Kraepelinian invisible college*' (Rogler 1997) of research psychiatrists who were in tune with the increasing medicalization of American society. Their attempts to systematize diagnosis through the development of agreed criteria ensured that the American view of diagnosis was brought into line with that of the rest of the world. This facilitated communication between countries and fostered considerable growth in psychiatric research during the next quarter century. Across the world of psychiatry it became clearer and easier to compare research findings and interpret the results of the burgeoning fields of genetic, **neuroradiological**, and **psychopharmacological** inquiry.

New psychotherapists and psychotherapies

Dissatisfaction with Freud had begun to appear from within academic psychology in the 1950s, with Hans Eysenck, Professor of Psychology at the University of London, leading the battle. Eysenck published data on the efficacy of psychoanalysis for neurotic disorder which suggested that it simply did not work (Eysenck 1952). Behaviour therapy began to appear as a form of treatment in the 1960s both in the US and the UK. Both psychiatrists and psychologists were involved in developing and promoting a range of treatments including **desensitization, flooding** and **aversion therapy** for a variety of disorders which included **phobias** (both specific and agoraphobia) and **obsessive compulsive disorder**. Around the same time, during the mid-twentieth century, a variety of other schools of therapy and counselling, notably the client-centred approach of Carl Rogers and the humanistic psychotherapies, introduced psychological therapies to a wider population. Most of these new therapists were not medically qualified and many had not formally trained in psychology.

During the 1960s leading psychiatrists and psychologists such as Aaron Beck (1976) and Albert Ellis in the US began to focus more on the *cognitive* aspects of disorder and to move away from pure learning theory towards cognitive science in order to try to provide more effective help for people suffering from depression. Many psychiatrists would learn the skills developed and taught particularly by Beck, but these approaches have gradually become much more the specialist realm of clinical psychologists. Within psychotherapy, some competition began to develop between psychotherapists trained in a Freudian model and those educated in the newer cognitive approaches. Cognitive therapy was quicker and demonstrated by rigorous research to be clinically effective and cheaper. The development of new therapies that were not only effective but demonstrably cost-effective in **randomized controlled trials** was particularly influential in the US, where Freudian psychotherapy and psychiatry were vulnerable in the new cost-sensitive environment of **managed care** because of cost and duration.

The second biological revolution

At the end of the twentieth century the position of psychiatry seems remarkably similar to that one hundred years earlier, with new promise of the answers to the causes and treatments of mental illness from biological research led by researchers such as Steve Hyman, Nancy Andreasen and Dennis Charney in the USA and Eve Johnstone, Tim Crow, David Nutt, Peter McGuffin and Bill Deakin in the UK. The last twenty years have seen enormous advances. The revolution in molecular biology has once again made psychiatric genetics fashionable, with progress being achieved for disorders where a single gene is involved such as **Huntington's disease**. The **psychoneuroendocrinologists** can now tell us a lot more about what happens in the brain and the adrenal glands (the **hypothalamo-pituitary-adrenal axis**) and how this relates to the development and persistence of depression. Evolutionary psychiatrists have even attempted to understand the evolutionary origins of emotions and mental illness (Stevens and Price 2000).

In psychopharmacology a wide variety of new and more specific drugs have appeared, replacing at last the older drugs with their multiple side-effects. In the last ten years, the drug treatment of depression and schizophrenia has been vastly changed. The psychiatrist is once again a prime target for the pharmaceutical industry. But the downside of this has been that the role of the psychiatrist as simply a purveyor of drugs has been reinforced, not least in the United States, with the arrival of **managed care**, as mental health care has been 'carved up' between the members of the 'provider' team according to who can provide evidence-based treatment at lowest cost. The psychiatrist is still the person with the knowledge and skill to do the prescribing. But even this may change as psychologists have sought to obtain prescribing rights.

Neuropharmacologists such as Arvid Carlsson (1996) have described in some detail what happens at the level of the neuroreceptor in depression and schizophrenia. The most impressive of all is the achievement of the **neuroradiologists** who, with brain-imaging techniques, have been able over the last twenty years to move from the early findings with CT scanning that the brains of people with the diagnosis of schizophrenia might show enlargement of the ventricles, to the extraordinary images achieved with magnetic resonance imaging (MRI). Functional magnetic resonance imaging (fMRI) enables us to see a response in the brain occurring as a result of some action such as movement or listening to music. For the development of magnetic resonance imaging, Paul Lauterbur and Peter Mansfield were awarded the 2003 Nobel Prize for Medicine. However, it is not known how the research made possible with these new technologies will actually impact on the everyday working lives of psychiatrists and, more importantly, the problems and distress experienced by their patients.

Lessons from history: orientation, faction or split?

What lessons can we learn from the history of psychiatry that will help us understand psychiatry today? Psychiatry is a medical speciality that specializes in taking the history of the patient, and yet few working psychiatrists today seem to have more than a sketchy knowledge of the history of their profession, and perhaps most importantly an understanding of the history of its dominant theories and creeds. Understanding the genesis of these ideas will give us a framework for understanding where the profession stands today.

Adolf Meyer in his book *Psychobiology* (1956) used this term to indicate an approach to psychiatry which considered a wide range of factors in aetiology:

> Each healthy person was unique and remained unique when ill; the psychiatrist had to understand his patients as individuals by understanding their biographies – it was not enough to assign them to diagnostic categories. (Gelder 1991: 426)

Building on his work, Anthony Clare (1980) and George Engel (1980) formalized the development of the biopsychosocial model, which attempts to bring together the biological, social and psychological elements of aetiology and treatment in a single encompassing model which has been informed by the insights of **general systems theory**. Anthony Clare, writing in the period after the assault on psychiatry by the anti-psychiatrists, argued that the medical model is not synonymous with the biological model but should encompass all three domains – physical, psychological and social. However, despite its emphasis in the teaching of psychiatrists, the biopsychosocial model, although received orthodoxy, may be difficult to discern in the everyday work of psychiatrists. We will return to a discussion of these issues in the coming chapters.

It should be clear by now that psychiatry is a profession which has been through considerable changes during its lifetime. Its members have sometimes pursued, often apparently single-mindedly, a biological orientation, attempting to discover the part that the brain specifically plays in the aetiology of mental distress. Leon Eisenberg has called this phenomenon 'mindlessness' and has warned, 'the peril is that psychiatry may come to focus exclusively on the brain as an organ and will overlook the experience of the patient as a person' (1986: 500). But at other times psychiatry has been dominated exclusively by those who discount the biological influence of the brain – a phenomenon Eisenberg calls 'brainlessness'. This view prevailed during much of the twentieth century in North America.

Not only do the biological psychiatrists of the end of the nineteenth century have much in common with those of the end of the twentieth century but, paradoxically, the pioneering doctors who created the humane asylums share many values and beliefs with those who later pioneered community care. In their book *The Perspectives of Psychiatry* McHugh and Slavney (1998) have demonstrated how the factions currently present in psychiatry can be derived from major themes of western thought present since the seventeenth century. Modernism, which embraces the ascendancy of science and technology and a commitment to rationalism, can be seen to have influenced psychiatry through the work of the great reformers such as Philippe Pinel, the observers and classifiers such as Kraepelin and even the psychobiological unifiers such as Meyer. The contemporary champions of modernity include the upholders of *DSM* and the reformers of the World Health Organization, but they also include the biological psychiatrists who seek to identify disease processes in the brain.

Post-modern concepts in psychiatry grew out of the development of phenomenology. McHugh and Slavney consider that Freud was the premier post-modern psychiatric practitioner because he believed that the emphasis by Kraepelin on formal signs and symptoms and on searching for the 'correct' diagnosis was merely a superficial form of psychiatry that detracted from the true study of mental disorders: discovering and understanding the source of underlying conflict. Freud certainly moved beyond the modernist assumption that mental disorders were products of nature and helped us to question the dishonesty and rationalizations of everyday life. But in attempting to free psychiatry from the rigidities of assessment and diagnosis, Freud and more particularly his followers developed a different form of straitjacket, another form of 'truth' that also could not be questioned. Psychoanalysts resisted research and dismissed anyone who questioned their particular authority.

From the 1960s onwards a third movement emerged, the anti-modern fundamentalists. They saw an authoritarian, uncompromising profession dominated by both modernists and post-modernists, neither of which was interested in listening to the patient. Within psychiatry, Thomas Szasz and R.D. Laing were the most influential of this movement, which rejected most of the received psychiatric wisdom. But, in throwing away what was bad about psychiatry, there was always the risk that they would throw away the baby with the bathwater. The challenge for today's psychiatrists is clear – to transcend the factions and splits, and devise an approach to clinical and professional working that draws from all of these traditions, respecting them, but at the same time trying to synthesize them into a coherent model of care. This is not an easy task. In the next chapter we will look at how psychiatrists are trained to do this today, and how they try and achieve it.

Notes

1. William Battie was one of the foremost 'mad doctors' of his era and a Fellow of the Royal Society. He was also a notable eccentric and appears to have lent his name to the second meaning of the word 'batty', which previously had only meant 'batlike' but now also means 'barmy' or 'dotty'. Possibly the original 'eccentric' psychiatrist? See Bewley (1998).

2. Milieu therapy is 'a means of providing an integrated, stable, and coherent context in which the optimal combination of specific treatments can be given to the patient'. Group meetings that encourage participation in information sharing, decision making and conflict resolution are a prominent feature – not as ends in themselves but as means of achieving a therapeutic goal (Campbell 1989: 757–8).

3. Women began to enter the speciality in the UK around the turn of the twentieth century. The first woman president of the Royal Medico-Psychological Association was Helen Boyle (1869–1957). See also Chapter 4.

4. Note that it was in 1815 that an Act was passed in the UK stipulating that the minimum requirement for any medical practice would be the Licence of the Royal Society of Apothecaries of London (LSA). Students without a university degree also began to take the exam of the Royal College of Surgeons of England (MRCS). In 1855 the British Medical Association was founded and the last part of the century saw the rise of specialist doctors and specialist hospitals.

5. There has been much debate about the cause of this rise in admissions. Recent case-note studies of records of large asylums suggest that the greater proportion of admissions was made up of patients suffering from organic brain syndromes such as General Paresis of the Insane (GPI, or the neurological form of syphilis) and alcohol-related mental disorders, while the proportion who might be given a diagnosis of schizophrenia was less than 10 per cent of admissions. This supports the sociologist Andrew Scull's hypothesis that the increasing admission rates could be accounted for by social factors and by the increasing public acceptance of the asylum as a suitable refuge for relatives with mental problems (see Beveridge 1995 and Scull 1984).

6. Hideyo Noguchi and Stanford Moore at the Rockefeller Institute demonstrated the presence of *Treponema pallidum* in the brains of patients suffering from General Paresis of the Insane (GPI – the neurological form of syphilis) in 1913.

7. Neurasthenia or 'nervous debility' is characterized by a variety of symptoms, notably fatigue, widespread aches and pains and insomnia. It remains a popular diagnosis today in some cultures (see Wessely and Lutz 1995).

8. Ben Shepherd points out that 'doctors of the PTSD generation have gone through the same learning process as the World War One doctors' and that there appears to be a 'recurring cycle with the war neuroses'(2002: xxii).

9. Postgraduate teaching in psychiatry in the UK is actually a very recent development. For instance in the UK the Diploma in Psychological Medicine was not established until 1922. London established its first Chair in Psychiatry in 1936 but Chairs were not instituted in most other British universities until the 1960s.

10. There were notable scandals at Ely Hospital (1969) and Whittingham Hospital (1972) in Preston, Lancashire (where I was, for a time, custodian of beds in an asylum). The inquiry at Whittingham followed the conviction of a male nurse on manslaughter charges, yet the official history of the hospital published on its centenary in 1973 (Makinson, 1973) plays the whole episode down.

11. This speech by Enoch Powell, then minister for Health, in 1961, is commonly known as the 'Water Tower' speech because of its reference to the water tower which was a familiar sight in the old mental hospitals.

12. The key ideas associated with R.D. Laing are critically reviewed by Beveridge (1998).These are (a) the experience of psychosis is understandable; (b) psychosis makes sense if it is considered in the context of disturbed communication within the family; (c) insanity is a legitimate response to a 'sick' society; (d) madness is a journey of self-discovery through which spiritual enlightenment can be achieved. Several biographies have been written of Laing. John Clay's recent book *R.D. Laing: A Divided Self* (1996), provides the insights of a Jungian analyst as well as being a very readable biography.

13. Life at Kingsley Hall was fictionalized by the American writer Clancy Sigal who spent some time there. R.D. Laing appears as Dr Willie Last. See Sigal (1976).

2

THE CULTURE OF PSYCHIATRY

At the beginning of the twenty-first century the profession of psychiatry is more closely aligned to medicine than at any other time in its history. The psychiatrist is a qualified medical practitioner, who specializes in psychiatry during postgraduate training, in exactly the same way that he or she might train to become a surgeon, a physician (specialist in general internal medicine), or a general practitioner. And yet for the patient, for fellow mental health professionals, and in the eyes of the general public there are extraordinary differences between someone who cares for the mind and one who can understand and repair the body. Indeed, among psychiatrists there are splits and disagreements between those who want to draw the profession closer to medicine and those who want to weaken the link.

By the time a young doctor enters psychiatric training, he or she will have spent at least five years at medical school, one year in hospital as a junior house officer in medicine and surgery, and possibly further years training, for example, as a general practitioner. Although psychiatrists are generally less conservative in their attitudes than other doctors (and indeed many regard themselves as more radical than other doctors),[1] medical schools are still failing overall to recruit proportionately from a broad spectrum of society (Roach and Dorling 2000).

In this chapter we will explore the culture of the profession and its representatives before moving in Chapter 3 to look at how psychiatry is both experienced from within (professionals and patients or mental health service users) and critically observed from outside. At the heart of this review must lie the assumption that psychiatry has its own 'culture' which has developed in western society over the past 200 years as a response to the forces and influences discussed in Chapter 1.

What is a psychiatrist in the twenty-first century?

According to the website of the American Psychiatric Association a psychiatrist is 'a physician who specialises in the diagnosis, treatment, and prevention of mental illnesses and substance use disorders'. The website of the UK Royal College of Psychiatrists further adds that 'psychiatry is a medical speciality that also draws on the social sciences, i.e. sociology and psychology'. This is an interesting addendum, because it highlights a conflict at the heart of what psychiatry is. Some psychiatrists ally themselves much more closely with the social perspective on mental illness than others. Similarly, there are some psychiatrists who ally themselves very closely with other doctors, and others who see themselves as closer to their fellow mental health professionals. Among those who ally themselves with fellow doctors there is a further potential split. Michael Shepherd comments:

> As a group the general psychiatrists sub-divided themselves into two broad groups. There were those who might have been general physicians or neurologists and there were those who might have been GPs or community doctors. The two groups were quite different in their outlook, in the way they approached the subject, in their thinking, and to some extent in their activities. (Shepherd 1993: 231)

Along another related dimension of attitudes to treatment, there are undoubtedly some psychiatrists, particularly those who have trained in psychotherapy, who still see the relevance of psychoanalysis to psychiatry today. Biologically oriented optimists see the psychiatrist increasingly feted as a physician who draws his authority from new knowledge of neural processes. Others, perhaps more jaundiced in their view altogether, consider that the real heart of psychiatry lies in its relationship with the mental hospital – the asylum powerbase of psychiatry for so much of its history: 'The modern psychiatrist is the descendant, not of the psychoanalyst, but of the nineteenth-century mental asylum keeper' (Littlewood and Lipsedge 1997: 10).

We have seen how this split between the biological and the psychosocial branches of the profession has developed over the last 200 years and how the pendulum has swung from biological ascendancy at the end of the nineteenth-century, through a century dominated by psychological and social approaches to mental health care, back to biological dominance (Eisenberg 1986).

Psychiatrists of a psychosocial orientation, however, have much more in common with the broader range of mental health professionals such as psychologists, community mental health nurses and social workers, who have appeared in the community during the last fifty years. Indeed, all psychiatrists in the twenty-first century work in a wide range of different settings, which include hospitals (both mental hospitals and general hospitals), but also settings in the community such as local health centres, and prisons. They also visit other places such as residential homes and schools. Almost all psychiatrists now work in multi-disciplinary team settings alongside other mental health professionals, but there continues to be a debate about the automatic right of a psychiatrist to be the leader of the team. As in other branches of medicine, psychiatry has also become more specialized. In the UK the majority of psychiatrists are general adult psychiatrists who may have a specific interest in one field of psychiatry, but are generally concerned with organizing and administering a psychiatric service for a specific population. However, in addition to adult psychiatry, a number of other specialities exist including old age, child and adolescent, forensic and substance misuse psychiatry, psychiatry of learning disabilities, and psychotherapy. A fuller description of the roles of each of these can be found in Appendix 1. Very few psychiatrists in the UK work entirely in the private sector, although, in common with other NHS consultants many do some private clinical work, or some medico-legal practice (see p. 66). An even smaller number of psychiatrists enter the pharmaceutical industry as psychiatric pharmaceutical physicians.[2]

How many psychiatrists are there?

Table 2.1 demonstrates the enormous variation in numbers of mental health professionals across the world. Each of the countries in this table represents one of the six geographical regions of the World Health Organization. Not only are the United States of America and the United Kingdom vastly better off in terms of numbers of psychiatrists than developing countries, but they also have many more allied mental health professional workers – for example the USA is particularly rich in psychologists, and the UK in psychiatric nurses. Yet these simple comparisons also belie geographical and economic variations within countries. In the USA most psychiatrists work in urban areas, and access is also considerably affected by the ability to pay.

Figures from England, reported by the Royal College of Psychiatrists (2002), show that there are just under 3,000 consultant psychiatrists in England, and just under half of these are women. About 88 per cent of posts are filled and there is currently a shortage of consultant psychiatrists in the United Kingdom (I will discuss reasons for this in Chapter 3) with a variable rate of vacancy around the country. The highest level of unfilled posts is in the north-west of England. It is not, however, just in the UK that there

Table 2.1   *Manpower data compared across six countries**

Compare by countries	United Republic of Tanzania	United States of America	Egypt	United Kingdom	India	China
Number of psychiatric beds/10,000 population	0.5	9.5	1.3	5.8	0.25	0.98
Number of psychiatrists/ 100,000 population	0.03	10.5	0.9	11	0.4	0.9
Number of psychiatric nurses/100,000 population	2	6.3	2	104	0.04	2
Number of neurologists/ 100,000 population	0.01	4	0.5	1	0.05	not available
Number of psychologists working in mental health/100,000 population	0.003	26.4	0.2	9	0.02	not available
Number of social workers working in mental health/100,000 population	0.04	33.6	0.1	58	0.02	not available

*Figures are taken from the interactive database of Project Atlas, available on the web at http://mh-atlas.ic.qc.ca.

is a problem. Even in the United States there is now recognition of a shortage of psychiatrists who are available to work in managed systems of care, or **Health Maintenance Organizations** (HMOs) (Goldman 2001).

Pathways to psychiatric care

Access to psychiatric care varies by health system of the country in which a psychiatrist is working. In the United Kingdom, the vast majority of psychiatrists work in the National Health Service. Only a minority of those people in the community with mental health problems will ever see a psychiatrist. The majority of people (more than 90 per cent of those with mental health problems) are treated by their general practitioners. The general practitioner is therefore the primary gatekeeper to specialist mental health care, in the same way as he or she is to other forms of specialist medical care (Gater et al. 1991). This pattern is found in other countries where general practitioners act as gatekeepers to health care, such as Holland and Denmark. However other routes also exist, for example via the accident and emergency department, or a police referral in the event of a psychiatric emergency or a person being found behaving strangely in the street.

In many other countries of the world the general population does have direct access to specialists. This has been the most common pattern in the United States, but is also the case in European countries such as France and Germany. Psychiatrists in these countries work both in private practice and in the hospital system. Many psychiatrists in the UK also do some private practice and have admitting rights to private psychiatric hospitals such as those of the Priory Hospital group. Access to specialists, however, is still usually via the general practitioner.

Where psychiatrists work as private practitioners, there has generally been less control over their activities by the state in terms of public mental health policy. However, with the rise in favour in the United States of the system known as '**managed care**', those who purchase care on behalf of their employees and the insurance companies who manage this care increasingly dictate how psychiatrists spend their time. American psychiatry has undergone somewhat of a revolution during the last decade. The pressure to cut costs has led to a growth in large **managed behavioral health organizations**. A patient who requires mental health care contacts this organization directly, and his or her needs for care are assessed by a case manager. Most mental health care is provided by non-medical therapists, nurses, psychologists and social workers, with the psychiatrist's role often being that of medication manager only. This contrasts considerably with the prolonged psychoanalytic treatment usually associated with the image of American psychiatry, and it has led to a considerable upheaval in the profession.[3]

Yet in other countries the situation is very similar, in that most mental health care is not in fact provided by psychiatrists. In the UK, when seeking specialist care the general practitioner today most commonly refers the patient to some kind of community mental health resource, generally a multi-disciplinary team made up of community psychiatric nurses, a social worker, psychologist, occupational therapist, with input from a psychiatrist. Managing this interface has become a constant preoccupation for mental health services (Gask et al. 1997). The problem is that many general practitioners and indeed patients would like more access to mental health services, particularly to consultant psychiatrists. However, given the shortage of psychiatrists and the sheer size of the problem of mental illness in the community, access to care is necessarily limited. Appropriateness of referral is contentious, and the patient, his GP and the mental health worker may all have differing views. General practitioners in the UK are provided with guidelines about who to refer[4] but the actual threshold for acceptance varies from place to place. In the inner city it can be difficult to gain access to the specialist mental health services unless you are psychotic, that is, suffering from **delusions** or **hallucinations**, and likely to fulfil diagnostic requirements for **schizophrenia** or **bipolar disorder**. Outside these areas referral is easier to obtain. However, guidelines for referral do not necessarily indicate whether or not the patient will actually see a psychiatrist. As in the USA, most care is provided by other mental health professionals and the role of the psychiatrist is perhaps less clear now than in the past.

A minority of British psychiatrists spend some time working in the primary care setting,[5] usually running an outpatient clinic based in the general practitioner's surgery, and/or attending primary care team meetings to discuss particular patients about whom the general practitioner would like some advice. This approach is called 'consultation-liaison' or 'shared-care' and is indicative of a trend towards integrating mental health and primary care that has been apparent in Europe, the United States and Australia for the last forty years (Craven and Bland 2002).

Professional organizations

In the USA and the UK the key professional organizations for psychiatrists have a long history. The Royal College of Psychiatrists started life as the 'Association for Medical Officers of Asylums and Hospitals for the Insane', but the title was later changed to the Medico-Psychological Association, and in 1971 to the Royal College of Psychiatrists. The birth of the 'college' was not without dispute given that there was a split among the senior psychiatrists of the time with academic psychiatrists favouring closer links with the Royal College of Physicians, while psychiatrists working in large mental hospitals, the asylum doctors, who feared that they would be neglected and frozen out from power and influence, favoured an independent college of their own. In fact, as has been pointed out (Clare 1999), since 1971 the institutional base of psychiatry has been eroded by the running-down of psychiatric hospitals which were once the powerhouse of the profession. It is now not only psychiatrists but others who work in the community as part of the mental health professions who lay claim to speak on behalf of the mental health sector and they have sometimes challenged the expertise of the psychiatrist and his or her right to be the leader of the team.

The Royal College of Psychiatrists in the UK serves as the professional and educational body for psychiatrists in the United Kingdom and the Republic of Ireland. Its stated aims are:

- advancing the science and practice of psychiatry and related subjects;
- furthering public education in psychiatry and related subjects;
- promoting study and research work in psychiatry and all sciences and disciplines connected with the understanding and treatment of mental disorder in all its forms and aspects and related subjects and publishing the results of all such study and research.

As well as running its membership exam (MRCPsych – which psychiatrists in training need to pass to move on to higher training and a consultant appointment) and visiting and approving hospitals for training purposes, the college also organizes conferences, lectures, and educational activities. It publishes a wide range of books and educational materials as well as its own journals, most notably the *British Journal of Psychiatry*. It also possesses its own in-house research unit, and a superb press office (Hart 2001), which makes sure the voice of the profession is heard in an increasingly competitive and political environment.

Nevertheless, debate about the proper *leadership* role of the college continues (Holloway 1999; Kendell 1999). The college does not negotiate terms and conditions of service, unlike such associations as the BMA, but has played a key role in upholding standards through its role in postgraduate medical education. Yet, despite its attempts, it has not been particularly successful at influencing UK Department of Health policy, perhaps partly because it is no longer seen as the 'only' voice speaking on mental health care. A questionnaire sent to a representative sample of college members at the end of 1997 indicated that its most significant failure in the eyes of members has been its failure to influence government policies for the treatment of mental illness. Professor Anthony Clare, responding to criticism that the 'scientific psychopathology' of modern western psychiatry had little to offer people in developing countries, has argued passionately:

> for the College to improve its support for psychiatrists and provide a better public definition of what it is psychiatrists do, of where psychiatry is going and should be going and how that journey should shape and affect not just psychiatrists and their patients but medicine and society, national and international. (Clare 1999: 2)

This is admirable, but while British psychiatry has been wrapped up in its own parochial concerns, it has seemed a tall order. The late Robert Kendell, a distinguished academic, former Chief Medical Officer for Scotland and then President of the Royal College of Psychiatrists, wrote clearly about the proper function of medical 'Royal Colleges' that control entry to the higher echelons of the profession through examinations (1998). No doctor trained in the UK can get on to the specialist register of the General Medical Council or obtain a National Health Service consultant post without completing a training programme approved by one of the Royal Colleges and passing the appropriate Membership or Fellowship examination. If NHS trusts ignore the college's demand to improve the standard of their programmes they lose 'educational approval' and cannot recruit junior medical staff. However, once a doctor is on the specialist register the powers of the college are considerably reduced and neither the consultants nor those who employ them need pay any attention to the statements made about clinical standards or minimum staffing levels. Kendell supported the view that the role of the college should be extended into the policing of standards of clinical practice by established clinicians. Such policing has now been introduced for all doctors in the UK through the process of annual appraisal and re-validation by the General Medical Council with the support of all the medical colleges.

The role of the Royal College of Psychiatrists is undoubtedly changing. When I discussed the role of the college with the current President, Mike Shooter, he told me:

> I think if you'd asked somebody in my position ten years ago what the college was for they would have said that it was about training, it was about making sure that psychiatrists were trained well, it was about accrediting their training, it was about examining individual psychiatrists to make sure they were confident in their training. If you asked me now I'd say that the function of the college still contains that but it's much, much more political, of necessity. I think the college now has to take a leading role in, euphemistically putting it, negotiating with government and other bodies to get better resources, better emotional space, better public image for the proper operation of services for our users and carers. (interviewed 2003)

We will return to discussing the nature of these political pressures in Chapter 4.

Across the world

Most countries in the world now have a similar professional organization for psychiatrists. The American Psychiatric Association, for example, like the UK Royal College of Psychiatrists, dates from the early part of the nineteenth century and the period of the asylum doctor. However, it was not until 1961 that the World Psychiatric Association (WPA) was formally founded, signifying a move towards an international professional identity. The 1950s, as we have seen, were a time of great change and development in psychiatry. Jean Delay, who with Pierre Deniker had discovered chlorpromazine, pioneered the establishment of the WPA with Henry Ey, another distinguished French psychiatrist who served as its first secretary-general. This was an important period for international collaboration because the World Health Organization had just published the sixth revision of the *International Classification of Diseases*, which for the first time included a section devoted to 'mental, psychoneurotic and personality disorders'. A few years later the American Psychiatric Association would publish the first edition of its *Diagnostic and Statistical Manual of Mental Disorders*. Every three years the WPA organizes the World Congress of Psychiatry, in addition to a large number of regional meetings. It has representatives across five world regions and attempts to provide representation for all member national organizations. It also has many different scientific sections which aim to increase international scientific collaboration in the profession. Today, it is also increasingly developing an educational role, particularly in developing countries, in collaboration with the World Health Organization. However, the role for which the WPA has become best known is the part it has played in responding to complaints about the political abuse of psychiatry (discussed in Chapter 4).

Training in psychiatry

Teaching psychiatry to medical students

In all countries there has been an attempt, under the auspices of the World Psychiatric Association, to standardize psychiatric training and improve its quality. All medical students receive some instruction in psychiatry but this varies considerably across the world and even between medical schools in developed countries. The World Psychiatric Association (WPA) and the World Federation for Medical Education have produced a core curriculum for undergraduate training in psychiatry (WPA and WFME 1998) and there is at least a recognition now that although the majority of those practising as doctors will not undertake any postgraduate training in psychiatry, many patients in the community, particularly those seen in general practice and in general medical settings, will have some degree of psychological distress. The psychiatry that is taught in the medical undergraduate curriculum, therefore, must be appropriate to provide an adequate basis for a large number of different specialities, and very specifically for the needs of the pre-registration house officer.[6] But what constitutes a core curriculum in psychiatry? What are the core psychiatric skills that all doctors should acquire? A recent survey of medical schools in the UK and Ireland (Ring et al. 1999) reviewed the core conditions and skills for teaching in the undergraduate psychiatric curriculum in psychiatry (see Boxes 1 and 2).

Box 1   Conditions thought by less than 85% of respondents to a questionnaire sent to medical schools in the UK and Ireland to represent core psychiatric conditions that medical students should be taught about (from Ring et al. 1999).

- acute confusional states and dementias
- affective disorders
- anxiety, panic and phobias
- conduct and emotional disorders of childhood and adolescence
- obsessive-compulsive disorder
- schizophrenia
- substance misuse and dependence

Box 2   Skills thought by less than 85% of respondents to a questionnaire sent to medical schools in the UK and Ireland to represent core psychiatric skills that medical students should be taught (from Ring et al. 1999).

- ability to communicate effectively with mentally ill patients of all ages and developmental levels
- ability to take a full psychiatric history and mental state examination
- ability to formulate a differential diagnosis
- ability to consider family relationships and their impact on individuals
- ability to perform physical and simple psychological investigations in patients presenting with psychological symptoms
- ability to assess suicidal risk

They agreed that it was important that students demonstrate a commitment to maximizing the social integration of patients with mental health problems and be sensitive to patient concerns about the stigma attaching to mental illness. Currently, medical students in the UK receive about twenty hours of lecture time devoted to psychiatry, in addition to a mean of about sixteen hours of small-group teaching. Students also spend time 'clerking' patients (taking a psychiatric history and completing a mental-state examination of the patient) and presenting cases to teaching staff. Use of problem-based learning strategies is growing but there is still a dearth of tutors who are adequately trained in facilitating small-group teaching. In psychiatry, as in other specialities in medicine taught in the undergraduate curriculum, there is a pressure to move away from overloading students with facts towards employing newer teaching methods. Compared to the past, medical students spend a lot more time out in the community with other mental health professionals and also have the opportunity to learn about psychiatry during their primary care attachments; however, this depends on the skill and interest of the primary care doctor to whom they are attached. Some research has suggested that male medical students tend to have a less positive attitude to psychiatry than female students (Wilkinson et al. 1983). There is no sex difference in performance at assessment but students from overseas do seem to fare significantly worse (Cullivan et al. 1999).

Many of those who qualify as doctors will receive no further training in psychiatry throughout their career. Nevertheless, approximately half of those who train in general practice do some further psychiatric training during their vocational training in general practice (usually six months). However, this is often not perceived as being relevant to the needs of a trainee general practitioner (Williams 1998) as it may be concerned with inpatient psychiatry and severe mental illness rather than with the commoner problems of anxiety and depression which are seen in primary care.

Postgraduate training

In most countries where professional training for psychiatry has been developed, this is overseen by a professional organization such as the Royal College of Psychiatrists in the UK. The World Psychiatric Association has recently also produced a core curriculum for post-graduate training (WPA 2002) although it remains unclear how training bodies around the world will respond to such guidelines for best practice in training. Further detailed information about obtaining training in psychiatry in the UK can be found in Appendix 1. Essentially, after five years of medical school training and completion of the pre-registration house officer post that is mandatory for all doctors, training can begin. Basic training, as a senior house officer then registrar, lasts three years and is followed by a period of higher training, in a specialist registrar post. Psychiatric trainees get experience not just of general psychiatry but also of the other specialities. Higher training may be in general psychiatry or specifically in one of the specialities such as psychotherapy or old age psychiatry. In all, postgraduate training lasts for six to seven years, then, in the UK system, the trainee is recognized as eligible for the Specialist Register of the General Medical Council and can apply for a post as a consultant.

With freedom of movement of professionals across national boundaries in the European Union, it should be perfectly feasible for EU nationals also to apply for consultant psychiatrist positions in the UK, as long as they meet requirements for appointment to the specialist register of the General Medical Council. However, it has been argued that the real European disparities concern style and content of training rather than the relatively straightforward issues of certification and duration of training (Neelerman and van Os 1994). French psychiatry has remained subordinate to neurology, and professional links between the universities and the asylums did not develop until the 1960s during the student riots when psychiatrists working in the asylums demanded separation of their discipline from the domination of neurology. Psychotherapy forms no part of the training of French psychiatrists, but is extensively provided for trainees in the Netherlands, who are automatically registered as psychotherapists on completion of training. Dutch psychiatry has generally been more concerned with religious and philosophical matters and clinical and ethical dilemmas in practice, and less interested in empirical research. The situation in the UK with respect to psychotherapy has recently changed (see p. 64) but the mandatory level of psychotherapy training is clearly still less extensive than in Holland. French psychiatry, meanwhile, still remains quite culturally isolated from the Anglophone-dominated scientific medical world and continues to use its own system of classifying mental illness.

In Britain speciality training has traditionally been longer than in Europe, and has been revised to bring it in line with the rest of Europe with one single specialist training grade. Psychiatric trainees today spend less time in 'service' work in the health service than they did in the past and have more protected time for training. Those doctors who do not complete their training to the level required to obtain a consultant post in the UK may obtain 'staff grade' jobs in the mental health services, but a significant number move around working in locum positions. In Europe there has been greater competition for training posts, which has led to an acute shortage of psychiatrists and a large number of uncertified but experienced practitioners. Such a climate of competition may also develop in the UK, but must be balanced against the *decreasing* recruitment rate for all medical specialities, including psychiatry.

Psychiatric training in the west for doctors from developing countries

An increasing number of psychiatric trainees in western countries come from developing countries. Some of these trainees are doctors from developing countries who have joined training programmes, for example under the schemes available in the UK, with the avowed purpose of returning as better trained psychiatrists (Tantam et al. 1996; Mubbashar and Humayun 1999). In practice, the vast majority of the trainees have been absorbed into the British health care system, which is currently hungry for recruits. But others who return seem to be disillusioned and frustrated with standards of mental health care in their own communities and therefore return again to western countries which they may perceive as having a more 'enlightened' regime of psychiatry. What is certainly clear is that western training does not prepare them when they return home for the wide variety of problems that they will simply not have seen during their training, including presentations of depression which seem unusual to western trained psychiatrists (perhaps with multiple physical symptoms), **catatonic schizophrenia** with a frequency much greater than in the west and other **'culture-bound syndromes'**. For psychiatrists working in developing countries, leadership skills are essential, perhaps even more than for the western psychiatrist, as he or she attempts to bring together the disparate community resources that exist and to achieve some kind of change in the system.

Kleinman (1991) argues that the real challenge is to try and create a combined clinical methodology that fosters both the treatment of disease and the interpretation of illness meanings from a broader anthropological perspective. Such a culturally informed methodology, however, would seem as relevant to psychiatry in multi-cultural Britain practised by native English-speaking psychiatrists or immigrant psychiatrists trained outside the UK as it does to the developing world.

The everyday work of psychiatrists

The Royal College of Psychiatrists' website provides a useful table charting the difference between a psychiatrist, a psychologist, and a psychotherapist (see Box 3 for my extended version of this). Most of the general public do not understand the difference between

---

Box 3 The differences and similarities between a psychiatrist, a psychologist and a psychotherapist (adapted with permission from the website of the Royal College of Psychiatrists)

Psychiatrist	Clinical Psychologist	Psychotherapist
Medical degree and further training in psychiatry.	Usually a psychology degree – may also have a higher degree (Masters, Ph.D. or D. Phil. usual now for clinical psychology training in UK).	Not usually a doctor – but can be. May also be a member of another mental health profession or have no such background – UK formal registration is UKCP (UK Council for Psychotherapy).
Can prescribe drugs.	Current debate about clinical psychologists prescribing drugs.	Can only prescribe if also medically qualified.
Broad expertise in diagnosing and treating mental health problems.	Broadly specializes in the way the mind works and motivation.	Uses talking therapies.
Six specialist areas in the UK General adult Child and adolescent Forensic Learning disability Old age Psychotherapy	Clinical psychologists can specialize in any area of mental health work.	Psychotherapists may specialize in particular therapies. Psychiatrists and clinical psychologists may also specialize in psychotherapy.

---

these professionals, but sometimes it seems to psychiatrists that other health professionals fail to understand this too, often interchanging the terms 'psychiatrist' and 'psychologist' in referral letters, apparently arbitrarily.

In the British National Health Service the role of a consultant psychiatrist (Dean 2001) may have more in common with the role of other medical consultants than with a psychiatrist working in private practice in the United States. There will also be considerable variation according to the sub-speciality of psychiatry practised. All medical consultants in the NHS must possess administrative and managerial skills appropriate to organizing their professional workload. They have to ensure that the service in which they are the senior clinicians is adequately managed clinically and adheres to the principles of clinical governance.[7] They all require the skills to be trainers and supervisors of junior doctors, staff from other disciplines and, in teaching hospitals, medical students. They need to a stay abreast of current advances in their particular field of interest and, since 2001, be subjected to an annual clinical appraisal and revalidation by the General Medical Council every five years. In addition to their NHS duties, consultants can also do private work, but full-time private practice outside London is unusual and doctors working full time outside the NHS will usually be employed in hospitals that are part of large provider organizations. Others will do part-time private office consulting and often have a medico-legal practice.

In addition to these broader tasks, psychiatrists in the UK will have specific roles to fulfil in their everyday work according to their particular interest and job title. For example, consultants in adult psychiatry are psychiatrists who are skilled in the assessment, diagnosis and management of mental disorders in adults of working age (normally 18–64 years). Adult psychiatry is distinguished from child and adolescent and old age psychiatry by the age range of its patients, and from the other psychiatric specialities by being the first and often only branch of specialist care to which mentally ill working-age adults without learning disabilities will have access. The general psychiatrist, in other words, is normally the first port of call for adults with the whole range of mental health problems. Some consultants in adult psychiatry will have particular expertise in other specialities and may, for example, spend a day or more per week providing a specialist service to which people with specific problems such as eating disorders or addictions can be referred. Depending on the size of the organization within the NHS for which he or she works, a full-time consultant may be available to receive referrals for patients with specific problems. The Royal College of Psychiatrists has historically recommended norms of service provision for consultant manpower. Currently the norm is for 4 whole-time-equivalent consultants per 100,000 weighted population aged 18–64 years.

Psychiatrists who work in large, public mental health systems like the NHS have two quite different roles to play, which Tansella (2001) has characterized as 'archaeologist' and 'architect'. Tansella's psychiatrist-archaeologist devotes his or her energies to understanding the symptoms and behaviour of patients in depth. In contrast, the psychiatrist-architect is more interested in *constructing* systems of care. In practice, psychiatrists throughout the world who work in public mental health systems will spend much of their time engaged in both of these activities, although there are pressures within systems, such as the emergence of managed care in the United States, that may at times push psychiatrists more towards administration than direct patient care. In the United Kingdom community psychiatry has been particularly concerned with the organization of mental health care systems and, as a result, has become caught up in the crossfire about the effectiveness of community care.

The other major source of conflict for the psychiatrist as 'architect' has been the ongoing debate about the *leadership* role of psychiatrists and challenges from other mental health professionals to the traditional right of psychiatry, dating from the days of the 'medical superintendent' of the asylum, to lead the multi-disciplinary team today. Many services are still professionally led by doctors, but clinical psychologists and mental health nurses are now also considerably involved in the management of mental health services. At the clinical level, psychiatrists perceive themselves (and are perceived by others) to have 'medical responsibility' for patients under their care (this is absolutely true for patients detained legally for whom the psychiatrist is the Responsible Medical Officer). However, the limits of this responsibility are unclear – which has led some psychiatrists to resist calls to increase the amount of liaison and advice work that they carry out, for fear of litigation. A better way to view the issue of 'responsibility' is to consider that all actors in the mental health team (and beyond) are clinically responsible for their own actions. Professor David Pilgrim, who holds a Chair in Mental Health at the University of Liverpool and is a leading critic of psychiatry and a clinical psychologist by profession, summed up the view of other mental health professionals thus in a recent conversation with me: 'Psychiatry retains its sense of slight aloof indifference: "We are slightly better than other people because we know more – because we are doctors and have longer training" and I'm not sure other mental health workers believe it any more.' (Interview 2003).

In the next section, we will consider in more detail the psychiatrist as 'archaeologist' by taking a critical look at psychiatric treatment, in the context of the biopsychosocial model, which has been particularly influential in the historical development of psychiatry in the UK during the last fifty years. We will also review the process of psychiatric formulation, which provides a framework for understanding how the biopsychosocial model is applied in everyday practice.

The biopsychosocial model
In his seminal book, *Psychiatry in Dissent*, written in 1980, Anthony Clare described the three different professional orientations within

psychiatry, which psychiatrists in training were required to learn in order to understand the aetiology, treatment and prognosis of their patients' disorders. The power of the biopsychosocial model was that it helped psychiatrists, particularly those in training, to make sense of the individual circumstances of their patients, understand the aetiology of their problems and plan appropriately tailored treatment. Clare was not the first to describe the model. As Pilgrim (2002) has asserted in a recent review, the biopsychosocial model refers to a position spelt out most clearly by George Engel (1980), who argued that if psychiatry aims to generate a fully scientific and inclusive account of mental disorder, then bio-reductionist accounts should be superseded by ones that adhere to the insights of general systems theory. Essentially, mental disorders, like other types of medical problem, emerge within individuals who are part of a whole system. This system has both sub-personal physical elements (the nervous system) and supra-personal or psychosocial elements (relationships, family, community and society). Engel asserts that attempts to account for mental disorder which refer only to the sub-personal, that is, the biomedical model, will not only be reductionist and inadequate in understanding the complexities of aetiology and treatment, but may also result in psychiatry being viewed as a dehumanizing profession.

However, as Pilgrim points out, these ideas actually stemmed from the original concepts of Adolf Meyer (1952) (see page 12) who was influential in British psychiatry, particularly for those academic psychiatrists and clinicians who trained under Aubrey Lewis at the Institute of Psychiatry in the middle of the twentieth century. Meyer's ideas were less influential in the USA, to which he emigrated, probably because of the enduring power of psychoanalytic thinking during the early to mid-twentieth-century. Pilgrim speculates that intellectual labour in psychiatry has often been carried out by émigrés of whom Meyer (Swiss) and Lewis (Australian) are good examples.

Anthony Clare's exposition of the biopsychosocial model came at a time when psychiatry was reeling from a long period of attack from anti-psychiatrists, and it appeared as a blast of positive, well-reasoned but far from defensive discussion of some of the key questions of the day. Clare translated for a more general reader the three different approaches to investigating patients' problems, understanding the aetiology, and planning treatment that the working psychiatrist needs to synthesize in order to be able to *formulate* the patient's problems (see p. 57).

The *organic or biological approach* lays particular emphasis on the role of genetic, biochemical, physiological and neuropsychological factors in the causation of psychiatric illness, and provides the scientific basis for physical treatments such as ECT and psychoactive drugs. In contrast the *psychotherapeutic* or *psychological approach* focuses on factors such as early childhood development and difficulties encountered during personality development. Treatment here gives particular emphasis to the nature of interpersonal relationships as seen in psychotherapeutic treatment. The third orientation, the *sociotherapeutic approach*, emphasizes the importance of the social environment, a patient's social circumstances, occupational status, family relationships and friends and the nature of the society in which the patient lives. Treatment focuses on coping strategies within the environments and the practical aspects of daily living. Clare went on to describe a further essentially *behavioural approach*, which is probably best seen as a second division of the psychological arm of the model.

The psychiatric interview

The initial psychiatric interview is a creative act. It is a study of movement and change. It is unique. The circumstances, the environment, and the people involved can never be duplicated. Even if the interviewer and interviewee wanted to replicate their own interaction, they could not; for with each sentence their relationship has subtly changed. With each sentence they define a new phenomenon. (Shea 1998: xi)

In psychiatry, more than other medical specialities, much depends on what happens during the interview with the patient. It has been noted that 'One often observes a greater comfort and intellectual curiosity in the discussion of the psychopathology of the patient rather than exploration of the interview process' (McCready and Waring 1986). The psychiatrist who interrogates the patient about psychiatric symptoms or psychosocial problems without considering the interview process in greater depth is behaving little differently from the surgeon or physician who interrogates the patient about physical symptoms. Both are adopting a style which will not endear them to the patient or ultimately assist in obtaining the best quality of information. So, whatever the psychiatrist's ultimate therapeutic persuasion, he needs to be able to communicate effectively and to possess the clinical skill required to carry out a high-quality assessment. Furthermore, the interview does not end with diagnosis. Whatever the treatment, it has to be explained to the patient and his or her co-operation negotiated in the consultation.

In psychiatry, the initial interview serves several quite different purposes (Rutter and Cox 1981):

- It is a means of asking questions to obtain factual information on historical events, happenings and activities.
- It serves as a stimulus to elicit emotions, feelings and attitudes.
- It begins to establish a relationship which will constitute the basis for further therapeutic contact.

During the **mental state examination** the psychiatrist needs to be able to clarify the nature of the patient's experience and get the patient to describe exactly what they are preoccupied with or concerned about. This means employing precision when, for example, asking about the exact nature of hallucinations, and when assessing the degree of suicidal risk. Clarification in the patient's own words is also essential when trying to establish the quality and severity of mood disturbance and when examining the nature and intensity of depressive thoughts.

Unfortunately, most interview skills training still focuses only on the psychiatric *assessment* interview. Formal psychotherapy training, a requirement now in the UK (see p. 65), may help to develop a trainee's pragmatic understanding of what happens in the human psyche and its relationships, but may fail to address the routine of the psychiatric outpatient clinic where the reality may be less contact time than the patient is already having with their own general practitioner.

Form and content

In order to understand the variation in the symptoms between individuals who may be diagnosed as having the same mental disorder, clinical psychiatry makes a distinction between *form* and *content* of abnormal psychological events. In his introduction to descriptive psychopathology (the identification of classes of abnormal acts), Andrew Sims clearly draws out the distinction and its implications for the doctor–patient relationship.

> The form of a psychic experience is the description of its structure in phenomenological terms, for example a delusion ... content is the colouring of the experience. The patient is concerned because he believes people are stealing his money ... . He is concerned about the content. Clearly form and content are both important but in different contexts ... the doctor is concerned with both form and content, but as a phenomenologist only with form ... the patient finds the doctor's interest in form unintelligible and a distraction from what he regards as important and he often demonstrates his irritation. (Sims 2003: 16)

As Sims remarks, the term 'phenomenology' has many different meanings, but in psychiatry it is used to describe a method for the eliciting of symptoms, as described by the philosopher Karl Jaspers (1913) in his early writings. The doctor tries to clarify the nature of the patient's experience, to understand it and feel it in such a way that his account of his findings evokes recognition from the patient. In psychiatry phenomenology is entirely subjugated to the purpose of trying to render the patient's experience 'understandable' so that diagnosis and treatment may proceed. The term 'understandable' is in quotation marks because it has a particular meaning in psychopathology. Jaspers distinguished between that which is meaningful and allows empathy and that which is ultimately 'un-understandable' which he considered to be the essence of psychotic experience.

The importance of diagnosis in psychiatry

Most psychiatrists consider the role of diagnosis to be central in the management of people with mental health problems. This is an important point of divergence with some other mental health professionals (Boyle 1999) – particularly many psychologists, counsellors and some nurses who view the emphasis on diagnosis as at the very least unhelpful, and even harmful because of the negative effect that labelling *may* have. Furthermore, not only has the systematic categorization of mental disorders found in *DSM-IV* assumed a central role in research but it has come to be seen as a valid indication of the real existence of discrete underlying disease entities. Arthur Kleinman reminds us that the positivist bias of most psychiatrists, brought about by the empiricist training of medical school, leads psychiatrists to believe that observations are direct representations of reality. 'Advances in effective psychiatric treatment of specific disorders and recognition that clusters of symptoms and signs have the same prognosis not surprisingly encourage the view that depression, schizophrenia, and phobias are "things" in the real world' (Kleinman 1991: 11).

Undoubtedly, *DSM* was a significant factor in making psychiatric diagnoses more comparable to diagnoses in medical specialities. The act of diagnostic classification is also implicitly linked with science; indeed Michael Shepherd (1976) has claimed 'To discard classification … is to discard scientific thinking'. In his essay on the importance of diagnosis, Kendell (1975) systematically challenges the arguments made by many psychoanalytic therapists and clinical psychologists that psychiatry should abandon diagnosis completely and substitute instead a lengthy formulation of each patient's highly individual predicament. He is adamant on the necessity of diagnosis to help us in considering which treatment will be effective, to communicate knowledge that we have learned about effective treatments, and thus to carry out research.

However, strict categorical diagnostic systems such as *DSM* are now widely used in clinical settings for which they were not originally intended – indeed a criticism of psychiatrists levelled by other mental health professionals has been that of a 'slavish' commitment to a cook-book approach dictated by classifications such as *DSM*. Critics of diagnosis have argued that the criteria for making a psychiatric diagnosis in the *DSM* are not theoretically based, and in many cases it remains unclear whether the dividing line denoting presence or absence of the diagnosis is useful, particularly when it requires the counting up of symptoms such as in the diagnosis of major depression or anxiety disorders. For many psychiatric diagnoses, the relationship between the pattern of commonly occurring symptoms to which the diagnostic label has been applied and the underlying disease process has still not been clarified, although a considerable amount of progress has been made in this field over the last few years. Mental health clinicians and researchers use the categories as a basis for defining the individual's problem, the likely cause of the problem, the expected course of the disorder, and the appropriate treatment to apply. In practice, however, this can lead to a simplistic approach in which biological assumptions about cause and treatment may be unduly emphasized. It is worth noting here that although Kendell argued persuasively for classification, he also stated that his arguments were in no sense of a denial of the value of the comprehensive formulation, and diagnosis by itself is never an adequate basis for treating an individual patient.

Alternatives to diagnosis, based upon a return to a broader formulation, have been proposed by a number of writers within psychology (such as Boyle 1999) but this has made little impact on current psychiatric practice. Although all psychiatrists in training learn about psychodynamic formulation this is rarely used in everyday working practice except by psychiatrists working in psychotherapy practice.

Bringing it all together: the psychiatric formulation

The formulation is traditionally the process by which the unique individual characteristics of each patient's case are summarized in order to try and understand the individual from the viewpoint of diagnosis and treatment and in biological, psychological and social terms. Although in everyday practice few psychiatrists will actually construct a formulation (and indeed a few biological psychiatrists may eschew the need for routine comprehensive assessment of psychological and social factors), the basic principles are applied in the construction of any comprehensive treatment plan.

The format that psychiatrists in training employ to construct the formulation is summarized in Box 4.[8] The descriptive formulation is a succinct summary of the illness. In the differential diagnosis, all diagnoses to be considered are listed in order of probability with the evidence for and against each one. It is crucially important to consider any current physical illness which might account for some or all of the patient's symptoms or signs. In addition to the primary diagnosis it may be necessary to consider a supplementary one, for example personality disorder and depressive illness.

Box 4   Brief summary of the 'psychiatric formulation'

- **Descriptive formulation**

- **Differential diagnosis:**
  - What are the possible diagnoses? List in order of preference with reasons for and against choosing each one.
  - Additional diagnoses (e.g. alcohol dependence and depressive illness).

- **Aetiology: considering *physical, psychological* and *social* factors under each of three headings – *predisposing, precipitating* and *maintaining* factors.**

- **Investigations:**
  - Physical: e.g. blood tests, CAT scan.
  - Psychological: e.g. score on depression rating scale.
  - Social: e.g. information from carer/family, home assessment.

- **Immediate management plan:**
  - Risk assessment.
  - Treatment – medication, psychological therapies, social management.
  - Information required by patient, family, team.

- **Long-term management plan.**
  - Risk assessment.
  - Treatment – including need for medication, psychological therapies, social rehabilitation.
  - Carers/family.

- **Prognosis: short-term and longer-term (for *this* person, with *these problems*, at *this time*)**

Under aetiological factors the psychiatrist will consider the detailed information gained from the history, particularly family and personal information. What may have predisposed the patient to the development of this problem? Were there any specific precipitating factors? Are there any important maintaining factors which may delay recovery? Why has this patient developed this particular problem at this particular time? The differential diagnosis and aetiology will inform any investigations that the psychiatrist is to carry out. What needs to be done in order to rule out alternative diagnoses? What further information is needed in order to clarify the aetiology? The treatment plan once again should stem logically from discussion of aetiology as well as diagnosis. Treatments may be categorized as physical, psychological or social and as short-term, medium- or long-term. Finally the psychiatrist will consider the likely prognosis, given the nature of this particular disorder occurring at this time in this individual.

Post-modernism and narrative approaches to mental illness

From the viewpoint of post-modernism the very creation of a diagnostic formulation might be seen as 'an arrogant enterprise, a self-deluding activity which convinces the psychiatrist that he has arrived at the truth about a particular patient' (Beveridge 1999: 574). The traditional psychiatric formulation is an exercise in trying to structure what is known about this particular patient. But it is only an exercise. Perhaps what is even more important is the process by which the patient's 'story of sickness' is negotiated and constructed between doctor and patient.[9] The importance of this narrative has become more apparent in recent years, with the renewal of interest in narrative in medicine (Greenhalgh and Hurwitz 1998). The narrative perspective is important as a way to understand the patient, help the patient feel understood, form a therapeutic relationship and begin to provide help to a person who is in distress (Roberts 2000). As time goes on, the narrative of the story may be renegotiated between doctor and patient, as one or the other begins to see things differently. What is important is that both doctor and patient agree on the plot of the story and, hopefully, can also agree to differ where they see things from differing perspectives.

Treatments of mental health problems: still a biopsychosocial approach?

In his review of the biopsychosocial approach in psychiatry, Pilgrim (2002) points out how it is tempting to describe the biopsychosocial model as an 'accepted orthodoxy', but how in his opinion this view needs to be resisted. Criticism of psychiatry continues both from without (from the user and survivor movement – see Chapter 3) and from within, with the emergence of a new professional dissent (postmodern and critical psychiatry – see Chapter 3). The strongest feeling within psychiatry is that the biopsychosocial model is being challenged by the emergence of a new biomedical orthodoxy powered by the considerable influence that biological research has had on academic thinking in psychiatry and on the teaching of psychiatry in universities.

There seems little doubt that psychiatric treatment involves more use of drug treatments than in the past, but a psychiatrist today has access to far more effective drug therapies than his or her predecessor fifty years ago. Few data exist on exactly what treatments are provided to whom today in British psychiatry. Such data are more easily available from the United States.[10] Psychiatrists in the UK will, however, generally be treating patients for whom treatment has already been tried in the primary care setting so the data is not comparable. But it seems reasonable to predict that most psychiatrists, perhaps excluding psychotherapists, will prescribe drugs.

Some will also prescribe **electro-convulsive therapy (ECT)**. ECT continues to be a very controversial and emotive topic. Many mental health service user organizations would like to see it banned. In the past there has been considerable concern about the way that ECT has been administered and in recent years a number of guideline statements (Royal College of Psychiatrists 1995; 1999) have been provided in the UK in response to troubling audit results (Pippard and Ellam 1981). ECT is probably used much less now than it was in the past, but it does continue to be a life-saving treatment for some patients, particularly those with a very severe depression who have stopped eating and drinking. This is why most psychiatrists continue to use it even in the face of criticism (Arscott 1999; Bracken 2002) and a sense, experienced by many, that it is nonetheless extremely frightening and inherently barbaric.

Although many psychiatrists will be trained in some form of psychotherapy, a significant number of these may feel unable to practise this effectively because of everyday time constraints. It is one thing to learn how to carry out dynamic psychotherapy in a training post, but another to try and do this in a routine general psychiatry outpatient clinic where the expectation is of rapid access and turnover of clientele. In addition, the psychiatrist may be only one of many mental health professionals trained in psychotherapy who are working in an organization. Indeed, other mental health professionals may be able to provide psychological therapies much more cheaply in terms of therapist time required. Increasingly, particularly in the USA, treatment is becoming fragmented, with psychiatrists providing the input required for pharmacological treatment and other therapists the psychosocial interventions. This may be one important reason for the demise of the biopsychosocial approach in psychiatric treatment if not in mental health care *per se*.

Perhaps it is not really surprising that doctors will retreat to a 'medical model', given the nature of their training. In *Psychiatry in Dissent* (1980), Clare fervently argued that the medical model should in fact be synonymous with a biopsychosocial model. Yet the model does appear to have lost some ground in recent years, with considerably less visibility within psychiatric texts over the last twenty years. To understand the probable reasons for this, we need to understand more about the growth of biological psychiatry, the current position of psychotherapy within psychiatry, and the rise of 'evidence-based medicine'. A final element, the pressures on the working lives of psychiatrists, will be considered in Chapter 3.

The rise of biological psychiatry

The paradigm shift from a psychodynamic to a biomedical and even neurobiological model of psychiatry has been greater in the USA than anywhere else. In the preface to her recent book *Brave New Brain* (2001), Nancy Andreasen explains that she has written about biological approaches to psychiatry for the lay person, 'to help them understand how the brain works and how it becomes broken in mental illnesses'. The language is stunningly seductive. Biological psychiatry is about seeing psychiatric illness in terms of how the brain works and how normal brain function becomes disturbed in the presence of illness. Bill Deakin, Professor of Psychiatry at the University of Manchester and a leading biological psychiatry researcher, explained it to me thus:

> I think schizophrenia is fundamentally a disorder of the social brain ... I see the psychoses as, broadly speaking, disorders of hard wiring. In the neuroses the wiring is fine but the volume gets turned up or the tone needs adjusting so you don't necessarily get sensible answers when you think about your self-esteem in relation to other people. (Interviewed 2003)

Despite the fact that such descriptions might seem over-simplistic to many mental health workers, they are often remarkably reassuring to patients and easy to understand. They also remove blame and have the potential to remove the stigma associated with mental illness by making it clear that mental illnesses are 'diseases' which are not caused by families or lifestyle. Nevertheless, they may come to be seen once again, as at the end of the nineteenth century, to be **degenerative**. Faulty genes may bring their own stigma as well as the promise of new therapies.

The early work of the new biological psychiatrists in the mid-twentieth century focused on the development of drugs. However, the current growth areas are undoubtedly **psychiatric genetics** and **neuroimaging**. Research at the interface between these is of particular interest, for example genetic differences in how drugs are metabolized. But in most of these fields of current research biological psychiatry has yet to deliver something that is useful to the clinician. Bill Deakin argues that it has brought us closer to understanding the pathogenesis of common psychiatric disorders but admits that much of this work is merely an elaboration of what Kraepelin knew at the turn of the twentieth century. Where biological psychiatry *has* delivered is in the field of drug treatment, and drugs that work on the brain. As Bill Deakin says:

> I think it's really important that I have ideas in my mind the whole time that I'm talking to the patient about which systems in the brain are going wrong … . I think in terms of neurotransmitters and what they do. This is a serotonin problem, what combination can we get to really push it? (Interviewed 2003)

Bill sees drugs as the most potent treatment that psychiatrists possess. There is little doubt that the everyday work of the general psychiatrist across the world is now much more concerned with the prescribing of drugs than it was in the past. And the pharmaceutical companies themselves have played a major part in achieving that.

David Healy, a psychiatrist and psychopharmacologist who has written widely about the history of the relationship between drugs and psychiatry, has postulated that in the discovery of the antidepressants 'what was to be seen was not an anti-depressant effect so much as the outlines of a disease – whose existence had been proposed before but which was now being revealed by a pharmacological scalpel' (Healy 2000: 56). This poses an interesting question about the relationship between drug treatment of psychiatric illness and the process of psychiatric diagnosis itself. Diagnosis is only useful in as much as it can help the psychiatrist in predicting what treatment will be effective. The drug companies meanwhile consider the results of trials of new drugs in order to find new markets for their products. Twenty years ago, no psychiatrist would have considered treating shyness with an anti-depressant unless there was clear evidence of a depressive illness. If this was a severely limiting function, referral to a clinical psychologist might have been indicated. Social phobia, as defined by *DSM-IV* (the fourth edition of the *Diagnostic and Statistical Manual*), is now an indication for treatment with an **SSRI (Selective Serotonin Reuptake Inhibitor)**. Healy has been a powerful critic of the drug companies (Healy 2000) for, he alleges, withholding evidence of the side-effects of the

SSRIs that emerged during their original trials. He has not been widely supported by other psychopharmacologists but he is not alone in his critical stance (Fisher 1996). No doubt he would point to the considerable financial support that the pharmaceutical industry has given to the psychiatric establishment, through sponsorship of meetings and research. The Royal College of Psychiatrists has recently moved to limit the level of financial support that it receives from the industry.

Interpreting the evidence base

In the opinion of John Geddes, psychiatrist and Director of the Centre for Evidence-based Mental Health in Oxford: 'Faced with the combination of rapid developments and increasing demands for information from patients, psychiatrists need improved access to high quality, clinically relevant information' (Geddes 1998: 337). With the increasing importance of biological methods in psychiatry has come the need to be able to interpret the findings of clinical trials. The first clinical trial in psychiatry was carried out by Linford Rees in Cardiff, who compared different treatments for schizophrenia – **insulin coma therapy, electronarcosis, ECT** and **leucotomy** (Rees 1950). The growth in trials benefited from the standardization of diagnosis discussed earlier. The current vogue for **randomized controlled trials (RCTs)** is not without its sceptics (see for example Healy 2001). Nevertheless, the psychiatrist in training today will need to learn how to appraise critically an academic paper describing the conduct of an RCT, and to understand the principles of systematically reviewing trials in order to assess the strength of evidence for and against particular therapies. The results of these reviews are used to write clinical guidelines not just for psychiatry but for every branch of medicine. Sources of information such as the Cochrane library of clinical trials and systematic reviews, in addition to the journal, *Evidence Based Mental Health*, provide psychiatrists today with a vast amount of synthesized data about the effectiveness or otherwise of psychiatric treatments. Evidence-based practice is also not necessarily in competition with the narrative approaches to mental illness discussed earlier. They are complementary – there is a gap between the empirical evidence base and the information that patients need and want (Szatmari 1999).

However, there is still a good deal of scepticism about introducing evidence-based practice into everyday clinical work, with 'clinical intuition' and the 'opinion of colleagues' seeming to be as useful in one study of psychiatrists' attitudes to evidence-based medicine

(Rees et al. 2002). Geddes notes that few psychiatrists have adequate access to good information sources and that psychiatrists' critical appraisal and clinical epidemiological skills are 'at best a little rusty'. Psychiatrists have generally been found to be in favour of clinical guidelines *in principle*, but there is little data about whether this actually translates into use of guidelines in practice and indeed any improved outcome for patients. Research into the effectiveness of guidelines as an intervention has been disappointing across medicine as a whole. Perhaps one of the problems with evidence-based medicine for the working clinician is that it devalues the aspects of medicine which cannot be easily categorized into testable interventions, the non-specific but nevertheless extremely important aspects of care.

Contrary to the opinion of a few biological psychiatrists, there is indeed a substantial and growing evidence base for the effectiveness of some specific psychological interventions – a fact that has led to increasing demand for mental health workers trained in these specific skills. Indeed the growth in evidence-based practice underpinned by a move towards managed care was one of the factors leading to the decline in the power of psychoanalysis in the United States. However, such an approach may once again lead to a fragmentation of psychiatric care, with different professionals delivering different interventions and an undervaluing of the central and key relationship that is forged with the patient. Developing this relationship, the therapeutic alliance, is one of the core skills of **psychodynamic (or psychoanalytically orientated) psychotherapy**.

Psychotherapy and psychiatry

In contrast to the United States, psychoanalysis played only a limited role in British psychiatry during the twentieth century. The biggest influence was in London, where there are still today psychoanalytically trained psychiatrists who practise *general psychiatry*, in other words they work with the full range of people who have mental health problems, including those with psychotic illness. Overall in the UK, about half of those who work as consultant psychotherapists in the National Health Service have had a psychoanalytic training, and there is evidence of a north–south bias, with the majority of psychoanalytic training in psychiatry taking place in the south of England. Today, the speciality training schemes in psychotherapy in the major cities encourage specialist registrars to have a psychodynamic psychotherapy but not psychoanalytic training.

Psychodynamic ideas, for example, about how to form a therapeutic alliance with the patient are respected by those even with a strong cognitive behavioural orientation or biological approach to treatment. According to Frank Margison, Consultant Psychotherapist at Gaskell House in Manchester:

> My experience is that if you make an over-strong case for psychoanalysis people react in quite a hostile and dismissive way and shift back into a quite rigid scientific paradigm; if you engage people in a conversation they are actually quite open and can acknowledge that psychoanalytic thinking is relevant to the broader field of psychiatry. (Interviewed 2003)

So what is the position today of psychoanalytic psychotherapy within psychiatric practice? Psychotherapy is undergoing something of a revival, not least because, after a struggle of over twenty years, training in psychotherapy has now been formally recognized by the Royal College of Psychiatrists as a core requisite for membership of the college, with a clear role in this task delineated for the psychiatric consultant psychotherapist (Royal College of Psychiatrists 2001). Undoubtedly, British psychiatry has been unusual in this respect, with psychiatrists from abroad surprised at the lack of requirement for psychotherapy training. The NHS review of psychotherapy services in 1996 (NHS Executive 1996) recommended that all mental health practitioners should have a basic training in psychotherapy and psychological treatments, but it was clear at that time that the majority of practising consultant psychiatrists did not measure up even to the minimum requirements of training proposed by the review and it seems unlikely the situation has drastically changed in the last six years.

Yet a number of basic psychotherapeutic skills are central to the everyday role of the working psychiatrist (Temple 1999). We have already looked at the importance of an interviewing style which is not simply a psychiatric interrogation. Much of the day-to-day care that is not easily audited for evidence of 'evidence-based therapies' consists of 'supportive psychotherapy', a much underrated skill that is required by all effective mental health professionals. Good supportive therapy involves the skills of listening, understanding, providing reassurance, shoring up rather than challenging personal defences and providing often quite long-term support for people who are considered to be unsuitable for more exploratory forms of therapy, because of severe personality disorder, major mental illness or simply lack of capacity to utilize therapy for one reason or another. The power of these 'non-specific' aspects of psychotherapy should not be underestimated, nor should the role that the personal relationship between the doctor and patient plays in the 'healing' process (as discussed by Kleinman 1991: 108) even where the doctor is using the latest, powerful psychotropic medications.

Yet there are also risks in these relationships for therapist and patient, including not only idealization of – or development of – undue dependence on the therapist, but also abuse of the patient, even inadvertently, by the therapist. All mental health workers, including psychiatrists, need to be able to assess these 'difficult' interpersonal situations. A period of training in psychotherapy, particularly attending a group to discuss personal reactions to patients, such as that described by Balint (1964), seems to help in developing both awareness of emerging problems and the skills for dealing with them. Without the skill to manage these situations, all mental health workers risk getting into professional and/or emotional difficulties (Rippere and Williams 1985). Mental health workers who do not work in a supportive team setting may be at greater risk of burn-out if they do not innately possess or have the opportunity to develop these skills.

The arguments for psychotherapy training in psychiatry have moved away from the debate about the need for personal psychotherapy of twenty years ago (Cox et al. 1982), which now seems to have fizzled out, to a clear definition of exactly what psychiatrists in training need to learn. This now specifically includes experience in a case discussion group, formal training in interviewing skills, and experience of being supervised in different therapeutic models and in both short and long therapies. But there is no doubt that old prejudices remain. Frank Margison says: 'I think psychotherapy is still the second cousin of psychiatry, still dealt with with a mixture of a grudging respect and mainly cynicism by most of my psychiatric colleagues' (Interview 2003). Jeremy Holmes, who has been at the forefront of getting psychotherapy back on to the agenda, has provocatively asked: 'Psychotherapeutic psychiatry – should there be any other sort?' (Holmes 2000). But perhaps this is a different sort of psychotherapy from that recognizable by the psychoanalysts. In his discussion of the biopsychosocial approach, David Pilgrim commented on how the central 'psycho' elements appeared to have gone missing in recent years. It certainly seems that pragmatic psychodynamically orientated psychotherapists have become more socially orientated. Frank Margison says (in his 2003 interview): 'People don't talk about Kleinian Object Relations as much as they did, instead they use attachment theory which has much more of a social orientation ... we have a much more socially orientated view looking at the life trajectories of people.'

This, however, presupposes that the patient is willing to go along with the doctor's view of what is the most appropriate treatment for a particular problem – or willing at least to enter into a negotiation about it. The final element in the psychiatrist's working life that we have to consider is his duty in relation to the law, and specifically mental health legislation.

The psychiatrist and the legal system

A discussion of the everyday work of the psychiatrist in many (but not all) parts of the world would be incomplete without a mention of the relationship between psychiatry and the law. The development of a framework of mental health legislation is one of the keystones of developing a national mental health policy (Jenkins et al. 2002) that has been promoted by the World Health Organization, particularly in the countries of the former Soviet Union. Some branches of psychiatry essentially become more involved with the law than others; the forensic psychiatrist, for example, will regularly have to write reports and give evidence in court. However, in the United Kingdom, most psychiatrists will have regular contact with the law through their responsibilities under the British mental health legislation (Mental Health Act – which differs across the countries of the UK). In England and Wales, detention in hospital on the grounds of mental disorder for a period of one month or more requires the assessment and agreement of two medical practitioners, one of whom is approved under section 12 of the Act as having a special expertise in the treatment of mental health problems and is usually, but not always, a psychiatrist. However, it was only in 1959 that compulsory detention was essentially made a medical decision. In many other countries it is the courts who decide if someone requires treatment against their will, not a doctor. Recent legislation in Scotland – but not yet in other parts of the UK – has sought to clarify the complex issues involved in determining the law in relation to patients who lack capacity to consent to treatment.

Psychiatrists and lawyers view the world in quite different ways. Jenny Shaw, a colleague of mine at the University of Manchester, is a Senior Lecturer in Forensic Psychiatry. She says of the judiciary:

> They tend to see us as quite woolly and grey … . We do speak different languages and they don't understand our language … . They try and force us into black and white [thinking] which is quite difficult I think … . On the whole they think we're a bit wishy-washy. (Interviewed 2003)

The psychiatrist who finds him or herself subject to cross-examination in court without adequate preparation can have a very tough time. But so also can the consultant who finds himself facing a particularly skilled solicitor representing a patient at a Mental Health Tribunal, at which the patient is appealing against detention in hospital.

For the general psychiatrist in the UK over the last twenty years there has been a trebling of the total number of compulsory admissions (or 'sections') under the Mental Health Act, a rise in the number of formal inquiries into 'untoward incidents', and increasingly complex legislation which is currently and controversially under review. Mental health policy is moving in the direction of psychiatrists assuming responsibility for a broader range of 'dangerous' individuals and having more responsibility for assessing risk to others. We will return to consider these themes again in Chapter 4.

Notes

1. Seventy per cent of a sample of British psychiatrists were agnostics or atheists and half of those who were politically committed supported the Labour Party (Toone et al. 1979). American psychiatrists were also found to be relatively left-wing and less authoritarian than other physicians (Rogow 1970). Both of these studies are quite old and it would be interesting to know if these findings still hold true with the rise in biological approaches to psychiatry.

2. According to Aitken et al. (2003), 731 physicians are registered with the British Association of Pharmaceutical Physicians, of which some 25 record psychiatry as their area of expertise. Their role includes both conducting clinical research and marketing support. Remuneration is notably more attractive in the pharmaceutical industry than in the NHS.

3. The literature is divided over the benefits or otherwise of managed care. What is certainly clear is that American psychiatry has been considerably challenged by it. For contrasting viewpoints see Detre and McDonald (1997) and Sabin (1995).

4. Guidelines on referral vary from service to service. General principles can be found in the *World Health Organization Guide to Common Mental Disorders and Emotional Problems* (WHO 2000). Essentially, if primary care treatment has failed or the person is suicidal or homicidal they should be referred. These are open still to fairly wide interpretation. Suicidal ideas are common in the general community and among those being treated for depression in primary care. In general, psychotic illnesses are managed by specialists, but, again, depressive or paranoid delusions also occur in severe depression which is not considered by some psychiatric services to meet their criteria for 'severe mental illness'. Diagnosis arguably continues to be more important than degree of disability in determining referral practice.

5. It is difficult to be sure about the exact number because the last national survey was carried out twenty years ago, but estimates have varied between one-fifth (Strathdee and Williams 1984) and one-third in Scotland (Pullen and Yellowlees 1988).

6. David Cottrell (1999) reviews the impact of the General Medical Council document *Tomorrow's Doctors* which has been influential in the redevelopment of medical education in Britain. 'Psychiatric teaching is clearly going to contribute to

core teaching in any new curriculum although it is interesting to debate what aspects …
might constitute the "core" if the pre-registration house officer is the reference point.'

7. The most widely used definition of clinical governance is the following: 'A
framework through which NHS organisations are accountable for continually
improving the quality of their services and safeguarding high standards of care by
creating an environment in which excellence in clinical care will flourish' (Scally and
Donaldson 1998). Part of the difficulty in implementing clinical governance is in getting the right balance between quality assurance (checking that a minimum standard
of care is delivered) and quality improvement (promoting the achievement of aspira-
tional levels of care).

8. What the new psychiatric trainee in the UK needs to know, including the
accepted method of psychiatric history taking, formulation and an introduction to
treatment and the mental health law can be found in *The Maudsley Handbook of
Practical Psychiatry* (Goldberg and Murray 2002). The practical utility of psychiatric
formulation is clearly demonstrated on a 'case-by-case' basis in the book *Making
Sense of Psychiatric Cases* (Greenberg et al. 1986).

9. Beveridge reviews the similarity between the work of the fictional detective and
the psychiatrist – the similarity between their work has often been noted in the literature but in the light of post-modernist theory the question must arise: are they both
misguided? They may be if they are looking for an overarching 'truth' but they must
instead be prepared to agree on and if necessary renegotiate the plot as they go along.
The mutually agreed 'story' may not be considered by the participants as representing an ultimate truth.

10. Data from a 1997 observation study of US psychiatric treatment carried out
by the American Psychiatric Practice Research Network (417 practitioners, 1,228
patients) are published in Pincus et al. (1999). Half of these patients were, however,
seen in a solo or group office setting so it is difficult to make comparisons with other
treatment settings. The authors comment that their findings paint a different picture
of American psychiatry from that portrayed in the contemporary media ('New Yorker
cartoons and Woody Allen movies'). Almost half the patients had a history of hospitalization and more than half were receiving anti-depressants.

3

EXPERIENCING PSYCHIATRY

How is psychiatry experienced by the public and practitioners? In this chapter, we will look at the way psychiatry is experienced, first by members of the public, who are greatly influenced by the media in understanding psychiatry, and then by members of the profession itself. What is it like to be a psychiatrist? We will also consider the views of other professionals who work in the mental health sphere, and the views of patients and those who use the psychiatric services.

Media depictions of psychiatry

For most people, including other health professionals, belief about what psychiatrists actually do has been governed by their representation on television, in films and in books. In a brilliant and comprehensive review of the 'theory and practice of movie psychiatry', Irving Schneider (1987) has shown how the depiction of psychiatry in films has developed its own characteristics, which only occasionally intersect with those of the real-life profession. His classification of the movie version of the profession certainly seems to apply across media depictions of psychiatrists in general. First, there is the familiar comical psychiatrist who is crazier or more foolish than his patients. This fits with the eccentric image of the psychiatrist that is shared by many other members of the medical profession and was immortalized on the large screen by Peter Sellers in *What's New Pussycat?* (1965) and on television by *Frasier*. The depiction of a group of young hospital psychiatrists as irresponsible and chaotic in their personal lives in the BBC drama *Shrinks* caused an outcry from the Royal College of Psychiatrists.

However, vying with this 'crazy' image is that of 'Dr Wonderful', who will go to any lengths in a deeply caring manner to help his patient. The best recent example of this is the role played by Jeff Bridges in the film *K-Pax* (2002), of which one reviewer wrote, 'a textbook illustration of Freudian detective work, which aims to get a malfunctioning character to go back into his memory and confront the long-buried original trauma'. The problem is that such a depiction of a psychiatrist at work is so grossly unrealistic as to be misleading. And Dr Wonderful always uses the talking cure. Indeed the majority of psychiatrists depicted in films during the twentieth century were psychoanalysts. Psychoanalysis offered a rich vein of psychological understanding to be mined in twentieth-century American culture. Films such as Hitchcock's classic *Spellbound* (1945), complete with dream sequences designed by Salvador Dali, established a link between the methods of criminal detection and the psychoanalytic method in the public psyche. Such has been the power of the psycho-analytic depiction of the psychiatrist on the screen that many patients still expect the typical British psychiatrist to have a couch in their office. In reality this is unusual even in the offices of those psychia-trists trained in psychotherapy.

Along with the crazy psychiatrist and the impossibly wonderful therapist we must have Dr Evil. His chief characteristic is his willing-ness to use what have been viewed as coercive treatments in psychi-atry including (too much) medication, ECT and lobotomy. Doctors of this ilk were seen in the films, *One Flew over the Cuckoo's Nest* (1975) and *Frances* (1982). But a much quieter yet still disturbing version of this doctor can be found in Patrick McGrath's novel *Asylum* (1997). Max Raphael's wife perceives him as a 'bloodless creature who behaved towards humanity like an insect collector, skewering them in glass cases with labels underneath, this one a personality disorder this one a hysteric' (1997: 123). In his most extreme form, the evil psychiatrist becomes a classic bogeyman such as Michael Caine in *Dressed to Kill* (1980) and Leo G. Carroll in *Spellbound*, characters capable of murder, or even the cannibalistic Dr Hannibal Lecter in the book and film, *Silence of the Lambs*.

Media psychiatrists
Although R.D. Laing was probably the first 'media' psychiatrist, the best known psychiatrist to the general public in recent years in the UK has been Anthony Clare, now Professor of Psychiatry at Trinity College, Dublin. In his fascinating series of interviews over the years, *In the Psychiatrist's Chair*, Clare has exercised his subtle charm on the listeners of BBC Radio 4. He is a consummate and intelli-gent interviewer who seems much more interested in the other person than in demonstrating to the listener his own talent. Latterly Dr Raj Persaud has become a ubiquitous commentator, not confin-ing himself to mental health issues only – which has led to him being lampooned by the media itself.[1] Yet though there are many within the profession who feel unhappy that Dr Persaud is now its best known representative, psychiatrists continue to be reluctant to raise

their head above the parapet. This is understandable, given that it is widely considered unethical to talk about one's own clinical work and unprofessional to comment on issues beyond one's area of expertise. Does raising the profile of psychiatry in the media necessarily mean trivializing the nature of mental illness? The answer should surely be no, but it is essential that psychiatrists do not run the risk of pretending that their expertise is much greater than it actually is.

The overselling of psychiatry in the middle of the twentieth century contributed to the problems that it has experienced in recent years. As Norman Sartorius commented:

> Psychiatrists were asked to draw psychological profiles of statesmen whom they had never seen and accepted to do so, although there is nothing in their trade that would qualify them for this task. That they are asked to do so is not their fault: that they accept that task is. Psychiatrists make statements – invited by others or spontaneously – about the psychological meaning of rituals in a cultural setting that they have neither studied nor are qualified to study. Psychiatrists write about 'political psychiatry' about the personality of nations, reasons for war and about too many other things. (Sartorius 2002: 196)

Psychiatry cannot cure society and psychiatrists do not have the answer for a wide range of social ills. But this does not mean that the 'social' aspects of peoples' lives are not important to the psychiatrist. They should be of the utmost importance.

Experiencing psychiatry I: The doctor's view

> I found that I was more interested in the patient as a person than in any particular specialised branch of medicine.

The reason given by Heinz Wolff, interviewed by Sidney Bloch in the book *Talking About Psychiatry* (1988: 180) certainly resonated with my own reasons for going into psychiatry, except that I would add that during my medical student training it was something that I found I could do, and enjoyed doing more than anything else. My experience at the Royal Edinburgh Hospital as a medical student made me quite certain that it was what I wanted to do as a career – and Heinz Wolff's basic textbook written with Roger Tredgold during his period at University College Hospital (and markedly psychotherapeutic in orientation) was a standard textbook for medical students in the 1970s (Tredgold and Wolff 1975). Reasons for entering psychiatry may be different now for young doctors exposed to the different, more biological orientation of modern psychiatry.

Surprisingly, however, there have been very few studies of what actually happens to students over time – specifically, anthropological studies of mental health professionals in training. An important recent addition to the literature has therefore been Tanya Luhrmann's masterful anthropological study of the experience of training in psychiatry, conducted in the US during a decade of turmoil in the profession (Luhrmann 2000).

Recruitment into the profession: the medical student experience of psychiatry

There is evidence that the experience that medical students have in psychiatry influences their choice or otherwise of psychiatry as a profession. Students at different medical schools in the UK have markedly different rates of choosing psychiatry as a career, with an average of about 4 per cent of students making it their first choice. The movement towards recruitment of equal numbers of males and females into medical school might have a positive impact on recruitment, as female students do seem to have more positive attitudes towards psychiatry and are more likely to opt for psychiatry as a career choice. However, recruitment into psychiatry in the UK has become more problematic over recent years (Storer 1998; 2002) (as indeed it has been to many other medical specialities). In the US there seems to have been a steady decline in recruitment to psychiatry over the last thirty years with the result that in 1994 only 3.2 per cent of US medical school graduates chose psychiatry, the lowest proportion since 1929 (Sierles and Taylor 1995).

The most likely alternative career for students who are keen on psychiatry is general practice, and many students who excelled in psychiatry in Manchester were found to have chosen general practice as a career (Creed and Goldberg 1987). Students can too easily come to perceive psychiatry as not only different from other medical specialities but also as somehow inferior. Jan Scott (1986) concluded, after a study of student views of psychiatry in Newcastle, that from the undergraduate point of view psychiatry seemed to lack a proper scientific basis and was too inexact. However this was not the only view. Many students seemed to be considerably affected by the experience that patients with whom they had been involved during their attachment had not recovered, echoing the view expressed by Ellis forty years ago (Ellis 1963) that 'the fact that 40 per cent of British hospital beds are occupied by psychiatric patients will never lead students to be interested in psychiatry as will some therapeutic advance which empties these beds'.

The new medical curriculum has introduced students to patients with mental health problems earlier in their career and in a wider range of settings. Ideally they should therefore be inculcated with psychiatric knowledge and skills at a time when they are more receptive to new ideas and able to see the relevance of their psychiatry training to the rest of medicine. There are however downsides to this approach. In a problem-based learning curriculum students need tutors who are themselves sensitized to the importance and relevance of psycho-social issues in patients who also have serious medical problems. Otherwise the opportunities for learning about mental health will be missed, and it is even possible that students will simply have more opportunity to acquire the negative attitudes of their teachers. There is also now much less time spent actually with psychiatrists in the curriculum. As a consultant psychiatrist said to me about the current teaching schedule at his University: '*We don't get a chance to get to know our students.*'

Students are taught that using sophisticated scientific tests is an important part of good clinical practice, yet until recently such tests have been unknown in psychiatry, and even now do not necessarily contribute to clinical care but remain research tools. Emphasizing the biological aspects of psychiatry, in an attempt to make it appear closer to medicine, has been one route to trying to interest more students in psychiatry. However, other approaches suggested by Jan Scott were the development of a pre-registration psychiatry house officer post, which has now been pioneered in Sheffield, and more opportunities for liaison psychiatry attachments in training. This might help psychiatry to seem more relevant to the rest of medicine. It also seems crucially important that students perceive that psychiatric treatment can indeed be effective, and that they get a chance to see and help people with common mental health problems in the community, as well as recognizing that it is possible to improve quality of life *and* help patients to achieve recovery, if not cure.

The trainee's experience

For her anthropological study of psychiatry, Tanya Luhrmann (2000) interviewed psychiatry residents on two different training programmes in the US over a period of years. She comments: 'Medicine trains its students by having them act as if they are competent doctors from their first days on the job. Although psychiatric residents are "in training", they are also acting – from the day they arrive – as psychiatrists' (2000: 26).

This is wonderfully demonstrated in the columns that 'Michael Foxton' writes occasionally in the *Guardian* newspaper. Foxton is (probably?) a pseudonym for a junior doctor who writes about his experience of training in psychiatry. Some people have been offended by his frank style of writing. However, rather as most junior doctors preferred watching the cynical realism of *Cardiac Arrest* to the sentimental drama of *Casualty* on the television, I suspect that most psychiatrists find his experience of training in the NHS today more realistic than any of the examples of psychiatry in the media mentioned earlier. Whatever the branch of the profession, the experience of training in medicine seems to have a dehumanizing quality, but it is not easy to cope in the face of constant demands and confrontations. The junior doctor's confidence is badly shaken by a patient who asks how long he has been a psychiatrist. His response is to feel guilty and helpless and he turns to a colleague for advice:

> 'Boundaries, Mike. Just document the non-existent suicide risk, increase the dose and get him out of the door as fast as you can.' 'Is this transference?' I ask lamely. 'I don't care what they call it. You're doing fine. Regain the control you need without being controlling. Accept your feelings but hide them and try to understand it later. And remember, just because he's a psychiatric patient that doesn't mean he can't also be a prick.' (Foxton 2002a)

What this also demonstrates is what Tanya Luhrmann calls 'the antagonism against the patient' which is perpetuated from medical and surgical house jobs through the busy years of on-call during junior doctor training. Junior doctors can very often behave as though the patient is the enemy. Driving this there is the difficulty of trying to maintain a sense of providing humane and sensitive care in the face of the resource problems facing the National Health Service (Michael Foxton puts it well (2002b): 'Bugger analysis: how do I find a bed manager at half five?'). There is also the fear of humiliation if an 'inappropriate admission' (for example a person with a known personality disorder who is considered to be 'manipulative' and trying to escape his responsibilities) is admitted to a bed and his presence has to be explained at the ward round. Junior doctors cope with the demands of all medical specialities by learning how to be emotionally detached. Psychiatry is not an exception.

Through her interviews with US psychiatrists in training, Luhrmann (2000) observes how psychiatrists learn to diagnose and treat mental disorders in the US system, which has taken classification in psychiatry to new heights of complexity. She describes how a young doctor she calls 'Gertrude' is initially uncomfortable with the lists and categories that she needs to know in order to make a diagnosis using *DSM*. Later, because of the way she has been trained, Gertrude acts as if she believes that psychiatric illnesses pick out real and discrete disease processes in the body. She talks about figuring out what is going on with the patient the way an ophthalmologist talks about figuring out if the patient has a corneal erosion. At the same time, her primary practical concern is with what medication to prescribe ... . (Luhrmann 2000: 49)

However, Luhrmann's most interesting observations come when she is comparing and contrasting how the residents learn in a biologically orientated unit when compared to an inpatient psychotherapy service (of a type almost extinct now in the UK). On the biological unit, she notes that doctors had more authority and the young doctors were not resented by other staff because there was 'no question – given the biomedical model of illness – that the psychiatrists knew more about the patient's problems than any other staff members did' (2000: 132). The ethos of the unit was to help patients understand they were very sick and to help them get better. The junior doctors learned not only about the need to adopt a professionally 'paternal' medical view in managing people who were 'very ill' but also about the importance of trying to explain to the world that psychiatric illness is 'real' and misunderstood. This was quite different from what they learned from psychotherapy. Here the emphasis was on the similarity between people who have 'mental health problems' and everyone else, and importance was placed on self-determination and taking responsibility. Luhrmann found that psychiatrists have to learn both medical and psychotherapeutic approaches to treatment and integrate these in one way or another, yet both models carry with them different assumptions about what causes mental illness, how to manage it, and how a person with a mental health problem will eventually change over time.

Psychiatry is straightforward when a person is starkly crazy, very psychotic. You know you cannot trust what he says about himself. A doctor knows he has to be in charge, the way a mother is in charge of her child and makes decisions for him (no ice-cream before dinner) that violate his wants and yet are better for him in the long run. It is easy to say that there is an illness affecting that person's judgment. But it's not like that, if a patient is depressed but says she's fine now and wants to leave, or, as this young man said, he thinks that psychiatric medication slows down his thoughts and he doesn't want to write his dissertation on lithium, how does a doctor decide who really knows best? Who gives the young psychiatrist the authority to say, 'you're more depressed than you think'? That 'you have an illness that impairs your thinking and so I cannot believe what you say'? (Luhrmann 2000: 138)

Psychiatry was one of the first specialities in medicine in the UK to offer well organized rotational training schemes to junior doctors.

Time off for attending courses to prepare for the MRCPsych exam is clearly planned into the training. Jobs are organized into training schemes across several hospitals, and these are regularly visited by representatives of the College to ensure that standards are being maintained. Losing training status can mean that it is extremely difficult to recruit junior doctors. One of the most important elements of training is supervision, recognized by both trainees and trainers as central to the training experience. Individual supervision in which trainees have an opportunity to discuss career plans, weaknesses and interests seems to be particularly valued. The nature of psychiatry, given that so much happens privately between the patient and the doctor, means that it is necessary to find ways to clinically supervise what actually happens in the consultation. As two psychiatric trainees writing about their experience of training said: 'No one except you and the patient really know what happens when you take him for an interview. You learn from your own mistakes behind the closed door' (Adams and Cook 1984).

The aim of supervision, through case discussion, one-to-one or in a Balint group,[2] possibly assisted by an audio or video recording of the consultation, is to try and decrease the sense of aloneness and increase the sense of competency of the trainee. The relationship between trainer and trainee can be inspiring. Most consultants can look back on certain trainers and quote the aphorisms which help them to get through difficult times in their day-to-day work.

Being a psychiatrist

The reality of being a psychiatrist, today, either in the UK or the USA, is quite different from those perceptions of psychiatry considered at the beginning of this section. Even those critical of psychiatry – and we shall look at these criticisms in more detail a little later – admit that it is a difficult and challenging job. There has been mounting concern about low morale in psychiatry in the National Health Service, particularly about general psychiatry. General adult psychiatrists work with community mental health teams in the front line of mental health care and there are concerns about levels of emotional exhaustion and burn-out of all professionals working in the mental health setting. Psychiatrists perceive an increase in administrative procedures, including the Care Programme Approach, and Supervision Registers,[3] which have encroached upon their time. There are pressures arising from requirements to achieve service targets relating to league tables, for example waiting-lists or number of patients seen. The number of official inquiries relating to incidences of suicide or homicide appear to some to fulfil a 'scapegoating process' in which mental health professionals are blamed, such that some have been asking questions as to the value of this system.

Raj Persaud has noted how it is not only patients but also psychiatrists who feel stigmatized today:

> It is almost as if while acknowledging they would rather see a doctor than anyone else when seriously ill, lay public and politicians also prefer practically any alternative, other than a physician, when determining who should decide how health care is delivered. Psychiatrists seem even more marginalised than other medical colleagues in public debate about practice. (Persaud 2000b: 284)

Experienced psychiatrists as well as trainees find it difficult to work in a system that is short of resources. They may find themselves in a position of responsibility without any authority over how the system actually runs or how decisions are made. The conflicts caused by trying to provide the best for your patient, when the system does not provide you with the resources for good-quality or even safe care have caused many psychiatrists, particularly those working in general psychiatry (who face particular conflicts that we will discuss in more detail later), to take early retirement.

Tanya Luhrmann notes some of the difficulties which lie at the heart of psychiatrists' relationships with other members of the mental health team:

> One of the difficulties of being a psychiatrist is that many of your skills, particularly the more psychodynamic ones, do not seem to be the kinds of things one needs to go to medical school to learn. Even the biomedical skills seem like things non doctors can learn. Psychologists, social workers, nurses know a lot about medication even if most of them can't legally write prescriptions. They spend more time with the patients than psychiatrists do … .
> Meanwhile psychiatrists are paid far more (after residency) than anyone else on the unit. It is easy for the rest of the staff to regard psychiatrists as arrogant overpaid extravagances. (2000: 132)[4]

Psychiatrists have moved out of the hospital, where they tended to congregate within their own department, and into community teams which are multi-disciplinary. With this have come both advantages and problems. For the psychiatrist who is capable and confident of his or her skills, clear about what he or she has to offer to the team which is *distinct* from the contribution of other members, and able to count on the support of both medical and non-medical colleagues, there are great advantages to be gained. However, in some teams there is difficulty in admitting that individuals do have specific skills to offer and a pretence that everyone can in fact do the same job. Psychiatry differs from many other mental health professions such as nursing and social work in that as psychiatrists are promoted to consultants they do not lose their 'caseload', or change to mostly supervising others, but on the whole *increase* the number of people they see face-to-face and have responsibility for. As Mike Shooter, President of the Royal College of Psychiatrists, said to me:

> We in psychiatry and medicine as a whole still have a caseload, for want of a better word, and I think we have to hold on to the skills that go with that. I think there's an allied issue here ... its one of the things that lies at the heart of demoralization in some areas for consultant psychiatrists and trainees, and that is I think we've become very unsure about what we're for, what our remit is and what skills we have as psychiatrists and doctors that are unique, or almost unique to us, that our training gives us and that couldn't be done by anybody else in the team, and therefore why do we earn our money? (Interviewed 2003)

Teams can be difficult places to work, fraught with personality clashes masquerading as interprofessional conflict. There may be a battle about who is the 'team leader' and wrangles about legal responsibility for care. These may be difficult to resolve. Workers from other professions, particularly mental health nursing and clinical psychology, may have different views about the terms 'medical responsibility' and 'clinical responsibility' from psychiatrists who tend to assume that the power and responsibility both belong to them:

> Who, after all, is the leader of the team? Legally, the medical responsibility is clearly at variance with the idea that any member of the team can be the leader, since doctors are legally responsible for ensuring the adequacy of any non-medical intervention including nursing and occupational therapy. This is even true where the interventions take place outside the statutory sector (e.g. in a mental nursing home run by a voluntary group). Such ultimate responsibility without authority is a recipe for anxiety, to say the least. (Thompson 1998: 406)

This view should be contrasted with that of a consultant reflecting (mostly) positively on her experiences in the development of a multi-disciplinary community mental health team:

> I was able to discuss my clients with the team, gaining from different points of view and improving co-ordination of care in complex cases where several professionals were involved. (Montague 1990: 19)

> To relinquish even a fraction of one's power and to share one's inescapable responsibilities as a doctor may be seen as threatening. To work as an equal partner rather than the automatic leader of the team

is an unfamiliar role to most doctors. I agree to work in this way because I came to feel that the team members respected my knowledge and experience of many types of mental health problems and their management. (ibid.: 20)

The difference between the views expressed above is striking. The first (Thompson) bears the stamp of the 'official statement' of a profession, defensive and conservative, but protecting the interests of the group; the second (Montague), the creative approach to team work of a confident but radical clinician of the type that innovates new services. But in the long term such a position may also become stressful and isolated. The reality for each member of the profession may lie somewhere on a line between these two points and may change over time. Undoubtedly many consultant psychiatrists in the UK system believe that having Responsible Medical Officer (RMO) status[5] means that they are responsible for everybody referred to the multi-disciplinary mental health team even if they have not seen them. But Kennedy and Griffiths, while asserting that 'even those professionals who question the pre-eminence of the consultant do not deny, and manifestly behave as if, the buck stops with him/her for the most difficult and dangerous patients' quite reasonably ask:

Are there really any consultants who have fallen foul of inquiries into serious incidents involving patients referred to secondary care whom they have appropriately never seen, nor been asked to see? (2002: 207)

In their view it is clear that psychiatrists who try and stick to the traditional role of taking global responsibility are likely to struggle, unhappily, with an ever-increasing workload.

Stress and unhappiness

Psychiatrists certainly do report higher levels of stress than other doctors, and higher work-related emotional exhaustion and rates of severe depression than consultants in other specialities, which is often given as a reason for wastage from the speciality (Guthrie and Black 1997). Jenny Firth-Cozens has explored the relationship between factors leading to choice of career and perceived stress, which suggests that the very factors that lead an individual to choose a career in psychiatry also make that individual more susceptible to stress (Firth-Cozens et al. 1999). This means that if we tend to screen out those who may be vulnerable we may risk losing the very qualities of empathy and sensitivity which many would consider key attributes for a psychiatrist. Bennet (1979: 184–5), writing about the concept of the 'wounded healer', noted that patients responded to the elusive quality of empathy which they perceived in some professional helpers with whom they came into contact. One of the circumstances that favours the development of this quality is 'the idea of the wound', by which he means that while most professional people keep clients at a distance some rare ones will admit, if not to their own weakness, at least to the possibility and potential of weakness. He points out that in many cultures it has been expected that the healer will also be a sufferer – which is indeed true of many who work in the field of the addictions.

Mike Shooter challenged what has seemed to be a taboo even among psychiatrists – admitting to having a mental health problem – by talking about his own experience of depression in an interview in the *British Medical Journal*:

> I think it has helped knowing what it feels like from inside. I don't foist it on them [the patient], but if I feel it is constructive to say to them, 'I think I have had an experience like yours for me it felt like this, I wonder if it is the same for you?' (Crane 2003: 1325)

Personally I have found that the experience of suffering from depression has enriched my experience of psychiatry and enabled me to understand how the other person is feeling about their problems, their illness and its treatment. This, however, has to be balanced against the impact that my work has, from time to time, had on my mood state.

Rippere and Williams (1985) discuss the interplay between the personal and the professional in case histories, two of which are of psychiatrists. A consultant psychiatrist describes how he became depressed when he was 'in the midst of an unimaginative, slipshod psychiatry and tortured myself because I could not put it right. I am surprised that I lasted as long as I did' (1985: 13). He describes what he learned from the experience. 'I brooded – it could hardly be called thinking – upon my plight as a depressed psychiatrist. There is no lonelier man' (ibid.: 14). 'I was bitterly ashamed at not being a tower of strength and I feared detection more than anything' (ibid.: 15). One of the contributors to Rippere and Williams' volume, who at the time remained anonymous ('Phoenix'), has since written a postscript and identified himself:

> Would I again choose psychiatry as my speciality? I think not. I would accept the misanthropic element in my personality rather than over-compensate for it by entering the most inter-personally demanding of occupations and opt instead for anatomy or pathology. (Jones: 1998)

There are particular experiences that can be exceptionally stressful for a psychiatrist. Working psychiatrists in the National Health

Service can expect, over the course of their careers, at least one and probably several patients in their care to commit suicide. Dewar and his colleagues (2000) surveyed UK trainee psychiatrists' experiences of patients' suicide and found that almost half of the respondents had close professional experience of suicide, with 31 per cent reporting that the suicide had an adverse impact on some aspect of their personal lives. The most commonly reported effect was a continuing preoccupation about the suicide and how it could have been prevented. Thirty-nine per cent recalled adverse effects on work, with increased anxiety and difficulty in making decisions, particularly when this involved patients with a recognized high risk of self-harm. One of the doctors commented: 'No other doctors are made to feel so personally responsible or guilty at having a patient die as a result of their chronic illness.' Another stress which is rarely spoken about is having a patient threaten to harm or kill the psychiatrist. It is extremely difficult to work out how common this is, although a survey in one region of the UK (Owen 1992) suggested that 34 per cent of psychiatrists had received such a threat and that male psychiatrists and those with less experience appear more likely to receive death threats.

Deahl and Turner (1997) have graphically described the pressures experienced by community psychiatrists in the UK: violence and the fear of violence, limited resources, overcrowded inpatient wards, problems of recruitment and retention within all mental health professional groups and a culture of blame. On top of this, policy that seeks to divert patients from the criminal justice system into mental health care places duties on psychiatrists to provide discharge planning, risk assessment and continuing care, but does not at present allow for community treatment to be compulsory. Any homicide by a patient results in an independent inquiry and a public report, which has added to the sense of moral panic increasingly associated with care of the mentally ill in the UK. There is also a sense, promoted by current health policy, that it is possible to predict the dangerousness of people with mental health problems more effectively and thus achieve a 'risk-free' society. We will return to discussing these pressures in a later section.

There are also other pressures that face all doctors. Concern over professional standards, fuelled by the Bristol Inquiry into standards of paediatric surgical practice, and increasing complaints about medical care have added to the pressures that doctors are feeling. There has been considerable concern about the rate of premature retirement of psychiatrists in the UK. In a recent study of psychiatrists' reasons for retirement (Kendell and Pearce 1997), common issues, other than ill-health and a real desire to spend more time on outside interests, were the increasing workload faced by consultants, changes in mental health policy and interference by management in clinical matters. Until recently it was possible for psychiatrists to retire earlier than other doctors working in the NHS, at the age of 55 with a full pension, but these rights have now been withdrawn for new entrants to the profession.

Not all psychiatrists perceive life as difficult and depressing as it is painted by Deahl and Turner but there is no doubt that general adult psychiatry in the UK is going through a difficult period. General adult psychiatry is the first point of entry for treatment, the 'showcase' of psychiatry. Medical students and postgraduate trainees get their first experience of psychiatry here. However, it is this subspeciality that is experiencing the most recruitment problems, as consultant posts appear increasingly unattractive and even unworkable. Many consultants feel unsupported by their colleagues in the other specialities. 'Some adult psychiatrists feel that they're being used as little more than sponges to soak up excess patients routinely referred to them from other psychiatric specialties – often without good reason' (Dean 2001: 13).

Psychiatrists are not alone among mental health workers in experiencing such stresses but they often seem to work in more isolated conditions with less peer support than do other professionals. However, in the study by Kendell and Pearce (1997), 47 per cent of consultants reported that their relationship with consultant colleagues was moderately or very stressful and difficulties with colleagues seemed to underlie some consultants' reasons for early retirement. This may be a reflection of the impact of cumulative stresses on interpersonal relationships between doctors, or simply illustrate that many teams, be they uni-professional or multi-disciplinary, are inherently dysfunctional! Staff sensitivity groups have been suggested as a solution to the problem of the dysfunctional team (see Haigh 2000).

Managed care – and NHS management

In the United States, managed care has brought with it a particular strain on the profession of psychiatry and has led to increasing dissatisfaction among psychiatrists (McKenzie 1998). In her account of psychiatry in the US, Luhrmann (2000) describes how managed care has been seen to support the biomedical approach to treating mental illness and led to a considerable reduction in the influence of psychotherapy. Under managed care psychiatrists have less autonomy. Insurers put pressure on doctors to reduce the length of stay of patients and discourage them from admitting the severely ill and the uninsured (Schlesinger et al. 1996). In many organizations psychiatrists have largely been reduced to checking medication, as other, less expensive mental health professionals provide care.[6] But as I found in my own research in a health care organization in the US, this is not just an unsatisfying job but also technically quite a difficult job. A psychiatrist explained to me, 'I'm really just there to manage medication; the problem is you can never just manage medication because they come in ... they've got psychosocial issues.'

Not all commentators, however, have viewed managed care with such suspicion. David Mechanic, who has been concerned about the failure of mental health services in America to provide care of sufficient intensity for the severely mentally ill while providing extensive psychotherapy to people with common mental health problems, sees managed care not as a threat but as an opportunity:

> to develop broader and better integrated systems of mental health management, to define treatment norms clearly and link them to a stronger evidential basis, and to develop performance indicators and better track the provision of services. Managed care also provides opportunities to train and use different types of mental health personnel and to direct them to tasks that were badly neglected within traditional mental health services. It has the potential of organizing services that were typically fragmented. We must remain alert to abuses of new managerial systems, but at the same time use this opportunity to guide change in constructive ways. (Mechanic 1999a: 166)

Mechanic's last comment, about abuses of managerial systems, has some resonance in the UK. We have not experienced anything of the intensity of the managed care revolution in the US, but what we have seen is an increase in the power of management within the NHS, notable in particular during the 1990s with the rise of managerial culture within the new NHS trusts.

Peter Bruggen, a retired consultant psychiatrist, interviewed many different mental health workers for his book *Who Cares: True Stories of the NHS Reforms* (Bruggen 1997). One of his interviewees, 'James', was a young consultant about to leave the NHS. He attributed the increasing untenability of his job not only to the pressures caused directly by the NHS reforms, but also to the changes brought about by government policy on mental health during the 1990s, and the resultant panic caused by fears about dangerous, mentally ill people wandering the streets (James called these 'Lions' Den' directives).[7] He, and the other clinicians interviewed by Peter Bruggen, found themselves increasingly at odds with management during this period.

They were patently instructed to recruit the user group, that is the patients and the carers and relatives, as allies in the battle. I pressed James harder. He described how on 'stakeholders days', when vociferous patients or relatives complained about psychiatric services, or said they wanted many more small units, the managers nodded strongly in agreement and later quoted them. On the other hand, when long-term patients or the elderly, or their carers, said they did not want be moved, their statements were dismissed as evidence of neglect or indoctrination by old-fashioned carers, and of bad treatment by psychiatrists in the past. (Bruggen 1997: 168)

Professional dissatisfaction with psychiatry

The changes in psychiatry, particularly in the US, have left many psychiatrists feeling unhappy with the direction in which the profession is moving. Doctors trained at a time when psychotherapeutic interventions were the norm to find the increasing closeness of professional organizations such as the American Psychiatric Association to the pharmaceutical industry difficult to tolerate.

Recently, it was dues-paying time for the APA and I sat there looking at the form. I thought about the unholy alliance between the Association and the drug industry. I thought about how consumers are being affected by this ... about the new medications, about side-effects and alternative treatments. I thought about how irresponsibly some of my colleagues are acting towards the general public and the mentally ill. And I realized I want no part of it any more. (Mosher 1999)

Antagonism towards the profession from within psychiatry has a long tradition from Thomas Szasz and R.D. Laing through to the current protagonists of anti-psychiatry such as Peter Breggin, a psychiatrist in private practice in the US, who has written widely on the subject and has been an adviser to MIND in the UK. His book *Toxic Psychiatry* (1993) despairs about 'purging psychiatry of psychology and psychotherapy', which he perceives as happening within the profession. He writes: 'If you've ... shared feelings and personal problems with some of your friends, then you may well have more experience and practice in "talking therapy" than your psychiatrist' (Breggin 1993: 20).

One particular new direction from within the profession has been the development of the concept of 'post-psychiatry'. Bracken and Thomas (2001) argue that in order to take up the challenge to adapt medicine to the post-modern environment as it applies to psychiatry, the profession must ask itself a number of questions:

- If psychiatry is the product of the institution, should we not question its ability to determine the nature of post institutional care?
- Can we imagine a different relation between medicine and madness − different, that is, from the relation forged in the asylums of a previous age?

- If psychiatry is the product of a culture preoccupied with rationality and the individual self, what sort of mental health care is appropriate in the post-modern world in which such preoccupations are waning?
- How appropriate is Western psychiatry for cultural groups who value a spiritual ordering of the world and an ethical emphasis on the importance of family and community?
- How can we uncouple mental health care from the agenda of social exclusion, coercion and control to which it has become bound in the past two centuries?

(Bracken and Thomas 2001: 726)

The post-psychiatrists argue that they are trying to move beyond the conflict between psychiatry and anti-psychiatry, not claiming that one or the other viewpoint is correct, but instead opening up the debate to allow a variety of perspectives to be deliberated upon. The approach argues that the voices of service users and survivors of psychiatric care should be afforded centre stage. In practice, despite advocating an end to conflict, its high-profile protagonists seem to be vocally antipathetic to the use of psychotropic drugs.

The post-psychiatry movement is probably better known to other mental health professionals, outside the profession of psychiatry, than to those working within it. However, its proponents have argued strongly that psychiatrists in training should have the opportunity to learn about this perspective on the profession. Duncan Double, a consultant psychiatrist in East Anglia,[8] has been foremost among critics of what he sees as the narrow approach to training:

A senior registrar in psychiatry, who had not long managed to obtain her first consultant appointment, once ruefully remarked to me that she had become 'irretrievably biological' in her approach to psychiatry. Although this is regarded as an acceptable outcome of her training, she was not able to deal with any criticism of psychiatry. It is reasonable to expect psychiatric trainees to be able to consider the ideological implications of their practice. (Double 2001: 23)

Many psychiatrists will recognize, and some will sympathize with, these concerns. There seems, however, to be little space and time within the profession today to debate such issues in the face of the requirement to fulfil both the day-to-day work of keeping the service going, and the juggernaut-driven modernization agenda of the British National Health Service.

The particular experience of women in psychiatry
Despite the fact that women are now increasingly represented in senior posts in psychiatry, there are still disparities between male

and female psychiatrists (Kohen and Arnold 2002). Fifty per cent of the psychiatrists in England are women, but only 32 per cent of consultant psychiatrists are female. However, women now hold 51 per cent of registrar posts which may reflect the increasing popularity of psychiatry with women trainees. Certain specialities such as child and adolescent psychiatry and psychotherapy are particularly popular, and psychiatry was one of the first specialities to promote flexible (part-time) training for women. Psychiatry is a speciality in which it is possible to find part-time work and/or job-share. Elaine Arnold is active in the Women in Psychiatry Special Interest Group of the Royal College of Psychiatrists and a consultant in old-age psychiatry in London. She commented, 'I think being a female psychiatrist is a lot easier than being a female surgeon.' She does not think that there is discrimination against women in psychiatry, and argues there is actually quite a lot of strength in being a member of a group which is increasingly important to the profession. The problems are more subtle. Women tend not to put themselves forward for higher training and academic posts and are more likely to get stuck in non-consultant staff grade posts.

Women certainly do not receive the same financial rewards as their male colleagues, but this is not because of discrimination in terms of appointment to consultant posts but because of failure to be as successful as male colleagues at getting the coveted NHS merit awards which considerably boost salary. They are not equally represented in academic psychiatry, and they tend to have a lower professional status than males. This may reflect, at least in part, the fact that men tend to finish their training earlier than women. There is some evidence that female psychiatrists experience greater stress than male colleagues (Kohen and Arnold 2002). Retirement because of ill health is higher and they do report poorer coping skills and more physical and emotional symptoms. Women doctors in general appear to have higher rates of psychiatric symptoms than their male colleagues and other staff working in professions allied to medicine (Wall et al. 1997). Among NHS doctors the risk of suicide is higher for women, which is not the case in the general population. (Hawton et al. 2001).

Ethnic minority psychiatrists in the UK

We have already considered the specific requirements of the immigrant psychiatrist coming to Britain to train in psychiatry. A large proportion of junior psychiatrists in Britain are themselves immigrants (although at the time of writing the Royal College of Psychiatrists is not publishing data on where trainees received their undergraduate training). Indeed it has been suggested that a greater number of psychiatrists in the UK are black or Asian than in the USA because of the greater prestige that psychiatry carries as a profession in the USA (Littlewood and Lipsedge 1997: 12). In the earlier part of the twentieth century psychiatry was associated with the Jewish minority, many of whom had fled Nazi Germany to practise in other countries in the west. However, psychiatry in Britain has become increasingly associated with other ethnic minority groups, particularly doctors from the Indian sub-continent. Many of these doctors were older than their British colleagues when they trained in psychiatry, some of them taking it up after failing to get jobs in other specialities. It has been noted that they are more likely to be orientated to a biological view of mental illness and they tend to be over-represented in the non-consultant staff grade posts, as their pass rates tend to be lower in the Royal College of Psychiatrists examinations (Littlewood and Lipsedge 1997: 12).

Littlewood and Lipsedge also comment that although, like many of their patients, the psychiatrists are immigrants, they find themselves defining normality and abnormality in British terms. They may have problems in understanding vernacular language and custom, and in acquiring a firm grasp of social and psychological theories that may seem entirely alien to them. Perhaps it isn't entirely surprising that in a speciality which requires competence in the subtleties of regional communication it is not easy to move from one culture to another, even if you have a considerable competence in the English language, as do many Asian doctors who are educated in English throughout medical school. Many trainees have an excellent level of knowledge and skills, but others are simply not prepared for the job, as one writer describes:

> Having chosen a field he is least interested to work in, befuddled by the terminology of dynamically orientated psychotherapy, perplexed by the anxiety provoking interview of an acute admission ward, lacking fluency in the English language let alone familiarity with the English culture and idiom, the postgraduate tries hard to put on a bold front. (Perinpanayagam 1973)

Trainee psychiatrists seldom complain publicly of overt racial prejudice. Nevertheless, one of my own (female) trainees has in the past experienced racial prejudice both from patients, angry and abusive at having to see a 'black' doctor, and from another consultant who was herself from an ethnic minority, albeit a different one.

Dinesh Bhugra, Dean of the Royal College of Psychiatrists and a consultant at the Maudsley Hospital in London, has direct experience of being an ethnic psychiatrist working in Britain. He told me he does not think that psychiatry manages doctors from ethnic minorities very well, although their representation at senior levels in the Royal College of Psychiatrists has increased in the last few years. He wanted to do psychiatry even from medical school, but at home in India:

> it was seen as odd for an Indian man to want to do psychiatry. It really had very low status ... Even when I arrived, in a place like Leicester, which has a significant ethnic minority population, there was only one Asian consultant, and only one SR [senior registrar] who was Nigerian. And after he finished his rotation he couldn't find a job anywhere in this country ... . There have been some consultants who are now retired, or about to retire, who have been in the system for thirty odd years and have actually survived, but there was obviously a glass ceiling .... Some of them obviously didn't really want to do psychiatry and they ended up in psychiatry because they couldn't do medicine or whatever .... There is also the biggest group which worries me the most which are the staff grades, people who did either their first part of membership and couldn't get through the second part [of the membership examination] doing staff grade jobs that no one else wants to do ... There is going to be a very interesting shift with the second generation [of immigrants] because they are not going to keep as quiet as people before me did. (interviewed 2003)

Experiencing psychiatry II: the views of other mental health professionals

Psychiatry has come to be used as a generic term to describe mental health care. In this book I have used the word to describe the profession of psychiatry, but many of those who are critical of mental health care in general do not make this distinction. This is unfortunate, but at the same time can be seen to be advantageous to critical professionals who do not wish to be associated with the mental health system. Take for example the introduction to *This is Madness: A Critical Look at Psychiatry and the Future of Mental Health Services* written by two clinical psychologists who themselves work in the NHS:

> In our society there is a system that claims to have treatments that can cure madness. It is something that we find even more maddening than a lottery-sponsored Millennium Dome. Occasionally known as the psy-complex [see note 9], more often referred to as the mental health system, in this book we have simply called it psychiatry. (Holmes and Dunn 1999: 1)

Thus it seems to psychiatrists that the brunt of criticism for the system falls on them even though they are not alone in trying to operate the system (although to many it sometimes seems like that).

Psychiatrists have a diminishing amount of power to change the system, as we have seen earlier. Two groups of clinicians have the most contact with psychiatrists in providing mental health care – nurses and clinical psychologists. All of these professionals most commonly meet together in the setting of the community mental health team.

The nurses' view

Mental health nurses work closely with psychiatrists both in the inpatient ward, but also increasingly in the community in the community mental health team. The traditional view of the relationship of the nurse to the psychiatrist has been one of 'handmaiden'. Indeed, in the 1980s many nurses were very pleased to have the opportunity to work in the community and develop their role as independent practitioners, receiving, they perceived, more respect and appreciation from general practitioners for their skills than from psychiatrists. Nurses are certainly perceived as being closely aligned with psychiatry, which is seen as holding all the power. But, according to David Richards, Professor of Mental Health Nursing at the University of Manchester, nurses approach mental health from a conceptual model – a psychosocial model, in which they are increasingly more skilled – different from that of psychiatrists. Many may resent what they see as their difficulty in escaping from the medical model. As one student said: 'psychiatrists brought the model with them and they still hold all the power ... the mismatch between what nurses believe and what they're actually required to do is such that it can never be resolved so long as mental health services continue to exist in their present form' (Jones 1994: 6).

According to David Richards, young psychiatrists tend to be much more cautious in their decision-making about degree of risk in community settings than experienced mental health nurses, and 'it can be a pretty irritating situation to be an experienced psychiatric nurse and have a Senior House Officer come in with power and authority and be clearly making quite inexperienced decisions'. However, the doctor has authority simply by being a psychiatrist, and will sometimes look down on nurses simply because of their profession. David comments:

Experienced nurses view most psychiatrists as pretty wet behind the ears ... I would view one psychiatrist as a personal mentor – others – you just hope never to work with them again ... . The thing that distinguished the psychiatrist who was a real leader for me was the fact that he trusted nurses – within an envelope of supervision and mentorship. (Interviewed 2003)

Yet, despite the common perception of medical dominance in the community mental health team, a recent study found little evidence of this. Community nurses seemed rather to perceive psychiatrists as resources with whom they could check essential things such as worries about medication or anything else requiring a 'psychiatric view' (Brown and Crawford 2003). This is a point of view with which David would agree. 'I don't think they are seen to have a leadership role – I think they are seen to have a consulting role.' What psychiatrists are seen to provide for nurses is their expertise in **phenomenology** and diagnosis and their knowledge of pharmacology. Yet, as nurses themselves become prescribers (and possibly even psychologists too take up this role – see below), there is a risk that this will become an uncertain area with the potential for interprofessional warfare.

Psychology and psychiatry

The relationship between clinical psychology and psychiatry is perhaps more strained. Historically, clinical psychology developed alongside psychotherapy as a discipline to carry out standard psychological assessments but subsequently its functions have extended and proliferated in the provision of psychological therapies, particularly **cognitive-behaviour therapy (CBT)**. Psychologists developed expertise in the treatment of neurotic illness, leaving severe mental illness and psychosis to the psychiatrists. However, in recent years, this division has become less distinct. The management of many people with anxiety and depression has moved to primary care and has become dominated by drug treatments. Nurses are increasingly involved in providing psychological treatments such as CBT, and psychologists are using psychological treatments in psychotic illness. They are also now much more involved in forensic psychology in the assessment and treatment of severe personality disorder, and there is a debate in North America (though not yet active in the UK [Birchwood 1991]) about whether psychologists should also be able to prescribe medication.

The problems of recruitment in clinical psychology are greater than in psychiatry with the result that many services are considerably understaffed. Many psychologists and psychiatrists work together very effectively. However, a sizeable minority of clinical psychologists are very critical of psychiatric care and the medical model.

There is a widespread misconception that a psychiatrist is a bearded man who asks you to lie on a couch and free-associate about your dreams while he offers Freudian interpretations of your remarks. This is actually a better description of a psychoanalyst in private practice. Medical training, with its emphasis on biology and factual knowledge, probably discourages more psychologically minded candidates from entering the profession. (Johnstone 2000: 131)

The same author, Lucy Johnstone, is critical that many of her colleagues do not speak out, appearing to feel that their 'interests are not best served by offending psychiatrists' (ibid.: 139). Nevertheless, much of the criticism of psychiatry has come from psychologists who reject current mental health services, with their emphasis on physical approaches to treatment, in favour of combating the origins of mental distress by tackling the problems of poverty, powerlessness, alienation and racism. To do this, they argue, will require much more emphasis on community action than on medical care, and a move towards a more widespread provision of talking therapies.

From the point of view of the majority of psychiatrists, there is no problem with this but they perceive psychologists as having opted out of the burden of trying to run the mental health care system, while still being paid from its budget. Many community mental health teams do not have any formal clinical psychological input, and psychiatrists and nurses tend to share the view that they bear both the brunt of criticism of the service and the major responsibility for running it.

Most critical among psychologists has been Dorothy Rowe, formerly a clinical psychologist in the National Health Service and a successful writer of self-help literature for people suffering from depression. As a psychiatrist, I find it difficult not to be offended, not to say angered, by her black-and-white style of argument. She has little time for those of us who seek to change the profession from within while at the same time continuing to provide a service and to get along with everybody:

As is the fate of all reasonable, peace-loving men, they get shot at from all sides. They talk about the importance of counselling and how psychiatrists must be trained in therapy, and the bio-psychiatrists tell them they are false and traitors to the traditions of psychiatry. They talk of the effectiveness of drugs, and psychotherapeutic psychiatrists pound them with facts about the dangerousness of drugs and the importance of life events and social conditions. And cantankerous psychologists, crusading social workers, uppity psychiatric nurses, and, worst of all, patients who call themselves survivors ... accuse them of being economical with the truth ... . It is all very sad, but it has to be said that they are the authors of their own misery. They should either acknowledge the implications which current research has for psychiatry or they should, like

American psychiatrists, resolutely stamp out all voices of dissent. Instead they just end up looking foolish. (Rowe quoted in foreword to Breggin 1993: xxiv)

The only research evidence that Dorothy Rowe seems to be prepared to acknowledge, however, is that for psychological treatments. As Bracken and Thomas (2001) state, it does seem to be important to try and move away from the sterile ground of arguing about which approach is likely to be effective as both have a part to play. It seems therefore a great shame that Rowe should be so critical of those who try so hard to find a way to make peace and adopt the centre ground!

On the other hand, David Pilgrim, a clinical psychologist and Professor of Mental Health, who has often been critical of psychiatry too, sees a mellowing in the relationship. He sees psychiatry as having become more demoralized as general managers have put new constraints on the medical profession, and this has

undermined the confidence and arrogance of psychiatrists. They tend to be more amenable, more personable and more ordinary in their relating to you ... . This has allowed psychologists to move back in to adult collaborative relationships with them ... . It's quite tough being a psychiatrist. (Interviewed 2003)

He is critical of the psychologists who wish to take up a more radical role as healers and opt entirely out of a system which they see as coercive. There is real suffering and need and a job to be done trying to provide care, sometimes for people who require this care to be provided within the framework of mental health law. The question of whether psychologists wish to take on the role of clinical supervisor under the new Mental Health Act in the UK has split the profession as psychologists have not, thus far, assumed such a formal role. But he does not see it as possible for psychologists to continue to walk away from the problem of dealing with difficult people with complex needs – many of whom require treatment under the law – leaving other people to deal with this.

Experiencing psychiatry III: the patient's view

I have myself spent nine years in a lunatic asylum and have never suffered from the obsession of wanting to kill myself; but I know that each conversation with a psychiatrist in the morning made me want to hang myself because I knew I could not strangle him. (Artaud 1947: 33)

The patient's experience of psychiatry can be accessed from at least two comprehensive sources, autobiographical and research into user's views of care. There are many examples in the literature, particularly the autobiographical literature, of people who have had mental health problems talking about their experiences of care. There is also both a research and polemical literature concerned with the experience of the patient or 'service user'. In their book, *A Sociology of Mental Health and Illness*, Pilgrim and Rogers (1993) described three distinct conceptions of people who are treated by mental health services.

- User as patient: traditional view where people are passive recipients of care.
- User as consumer: professionals acknowledge the right of consumers to express views.
- User as 'survivor': users campaigning collectively as a new social movement.

Several years ago I reviewed the autobiographical literature on mental health and illness and argued that it was crucially important for psychiatrists to listen to what their patients had to say about experiencing both illness and its treatment. This was so that they might understand how to try to bridge the gap that was opening up between what psychiatry was offering in terms of advances in biological treatments, and what patients wanted – which was frequently more opportunity for talking treatments (Gask 1997).

Sylvia Plath's strongly autobiographical novel *The Bell Jar* was published a month before her suicide in 1963. In this extract, she captures the (for her frustrating) experience of seeing a psychoanalytically trained psychiatrist in the America of the 1950s:

> I had imagined a kind, ugly, intuitive man looking up and saying 'Ah!' in an encouraging way, as if he could see something I couldn't, and then I would find words to tell him how I was so scared, as if I were being stuffed farther and farther into a black airless sack with no way out.
>
> Then he would lean back in his chair and match the tips of his fingers together in a little steeple and tell me why I couldn't sleep and why I couldn't read and why I couldn't eat and why everything people did seemed so silly, because they only died in the end.
>
> And then, I thought, he would help me, step by step, to be myself again. But Doctor Gordon wasn't like that at all. He was young and good-looking and I could see right away he was conceited. (Plath 1963: 135–6)

Doctor Gordon, in the usual manner of an analyst, says very little.

In his autobiographical account of suffering from depression, and experiencing the suicide of his mother, Tim Lott (1996) graphically described what happened in the outpatient clinic when he was referred to a psychiatrist. As is usually the case in a training clinic he initially saw the trainee who 'takes the history' before going to discuss the case with the consultant. Both will then usually see the patient together. This is probably the most efficient way of training, and, as Michael Foxton has demonstrated in his articles, psychiatry is no different from the rest of medicine in that new recruits are thrown in at the deep end and treated as 'psychiatrists' from their first day in post. However, it is difficult for patients to understand why they are not seeing a 'specialist' (and often of great annoyance to GPs who want a 'consultant' opinion). Lott was unhappy about this and not at all easy to interview – by his own account. Then he overheard the consultant say to the anxious trainee through the closed door of the consulting room: 'The intelligent ones are the worst. You have to be firm' (1996: 244).

Fiona Shaw, suffering from post-natal depression, vividly describes her first encounter with the consultant psychiatrist, whom she calls Dr A, after her admission to an inpatient ward:

> Dr A, my psychiatrist, arrived unannounced, a day or so after my arrival. She sat down opposite me and started asking questions. I liked her but was daunted by her. She was intelligent, with her own kind of wit, but never before had I met another woman on such unequal terms: severely depressed patient meets consultant psychiatrist. Her self-confidence was palpable from the first, while my self-esteem had by now entirely gone. (Shaw 1997: 41)

Stuart Sutherland (1995), a distinguished academic psychologist, writing about his inpatient treatment expresses the unhappiness that many patients experience, that they simply do not see enough of the doctors who are making decisions about them. His description of the boredom, frustration and pain of inpatient care, and health professionals' often quite amateurish attempts at providing psychological help is more enlightening than many accounts from survey research, simply because of the clear and concise language in which it is expressed. Similarly, William Styron (1992), a writer who has suffered from severe episodes of depression, is able to convey his anger and distaste at the psychiatric treatment offered to him – both psychoanalytic and biological. Ultimately, he is positive about the impact of drug treatment, but not uncritical of the manner in which it is provided. Of the advice offered to him by a biological psychiatrist he says: 'His platitudes were not Christian but, almost as ineffective, dicta drawn straight from the pages of *The Diagnostic and Statistical Manual of the American Psychiatric Association*' (1992: 53).

But not all of the experiences are negative. Elizabeth Wurtzel struggled to find a psychiatrist in whom she had faith, and she acknowledges the role 'Dr Sterling' played in keeping her alive over a considerable period of time. After she has taken an overdose, her psychiatrist takes her to the emergency room:

'I've never lost a patient before,' Dr Sterling says. 'I'm not going to start now.' 'Well I hope you're not doing this for the sake of your statistics.' And then I realise what a horrible thing that is to say to her. She has visited me in the infirmary, she's taken my phone calls at 3.00 am and now she's driving me to the emergency room, and the only reason she's done any of that is because she cares. (Wurtzel 1995: 283)

Researching the patient's view
However, there is another literature, which has been highly influential in the development of the **service user** movement in the UK. Large-scale studies of what people have experienced in mental health care and what they perceive as helpful may not always have been welcomed by psychiatrists, but nonetheless provide a valid point of view. Since the 1970s the mental health service user movement has become increasingly influential in helping people with mental health problems develop alternative ways of thinking about their lives and achieve changes in the services that they receive (including the promotion of complementary therapies such as in the Mental Health Foundation's *Strategies for Living* (2000)), and, in addition, to critique the existing mental health care system. Large organizations with a longer history, such as MIND (the National Association for Mental Health) and newer national alliances of individual **service users**, such as Survivors Speak Out, have been influential in shaping mental health policy.

It is clear that, whatever their views about psychiatry, people with mental health problems do not wish to be talked of by psychiatrists in terms of their diagnoses. They do not like the way in which psychiatrists talk about them as schizophrenics or manic depressives. This view was supported by Norman Sartorius (2002), one of the world's leading psychiatrists, when he commented on the way in which psychiatrists themselves are responsible for stigmatizing patients. 'There would be uproar if people suffering from pneumonia were to be called pneumonics and then prevented from obtaining driving licences because they might begin to cough and lose control of their vehicle' (2002: 65).

The 'People First' project conducted by Anne Rogers and her colleagues (1993) for MIND used qualitative and quantitative methods to try to understand the views that patients had of mental health care. As part of this project, people using services gave their opinions of the psychiatric care that they had received. Only about 5 per cent of those asked about frequency of contact with consultants during inpatient care reported seeing their consultant alone daily, and weekly contact was experienced by fewer than 40 per cent of respondents. However, patients reported seeing more of their psychiatrists in a three-month period when they were out of hospital, than when they were in.[10] Fewer than one-third of respondents reported interview times of more than twenty minutes with their consultants. Only half of the respondents thought that psychiatrists were easy to talk to. A similar picture emerged of the helpfulness of psychiatrists, with 54.7 per cent reporting that they were 'helpful' or 'very helpful'. About a third were satisfied with the explanation given by psychiatrists about their condition, and about 20 per cent with the information they were given about treatment. The qualitative interviews conducted highlighted examples of good and bad practice:

> They understand my problems and they have always given me an appointment when I asked for one. (Rogers et al. 1993: 48)

> It took many years for them to discuss properly with me my illness, diagnosis and medication. But now they have done so it has been very helpful. They are always there if I need them. (ibid.: 48)

> They appear unconcerned about the problem. They come across as being more interested in what they have to say about the problem than what the patient has to say. (ibid.: 49)

Psychiatrists who were disliked were reported as being distant and uninvolved in a helping relationship:

> They are passive. They don't provide any information regarding prognosis, diagnosis and treatment. They appear to be unimaginative and unsympathetic. (ibid.: 49)

> Reserved, detached, godly. (ibid.: 49)

> Condescending, complacent benevolence. (ibid.: 49)

Commenting on these findings, Rogers and her colleagues point to the gap between public expectations of what psychiatric care will involve. People think this will involve the psychiatrist paying heed to the patients' biography at length. However, in practice, after the first assessment biological treatments require a fairly brief interview in which the patient's symptoms are elicited and progress assessed. There is not necessarily an opportunity or even recognition of the need for a shared exploration of problems.

Persaud and Meux (1990) asked patients, who had participated in professional examinations for psychiatrists by allowing themselves to be interviewed, what they most valued in psychiatrists:

Almost invariably what the patients looked for seemed at variance with those qualities obviously assessed by the examination. For example, only one mentioned 'knowledge' while only one other valued 'experience'. The ability to listen was mentioned by eight (38%), while a further five included listening 'sympathetically'. One was less demanding and only required the ability to 'appear as though listening'. (Persaud and Meux 1990)

The last two decades have seen a wide variety of forms of user involvement in mental health services – ranging through information to consultation and control – arise in Britain (Campbell 1996; Peck et al. 2002). Some of these groups have drawn on ideas from anti-psychiatry, others have been influenced by the consciousness-raising approaches adopted by civil rights movements in the USA. Campbell comments that:

Antipsychiatry has become a slogan that is routinely used by traditional mental health workers to denigrate and dismiss ideas that threaten their expert world-view and status. As a result, some survivors are starting to talk of a 'post-psychiatric' approach. (Campbell 1996: 221)

The views of 'survivors' of mental health services can be potentially threatening and painful. But they cannot be ignored or simply written off as 'unrepresentative'. It is impossible to listen to people active in the user movement without becoming very quickly aware that many people have had unsatisfactory experiences of psychiatry. The development of the user movement poses a significant challenge to a psychiatric world that in many ways continues to look inwards to strengthening its own 'scientific' base rather than outwards towards exploring, reconsidering and possibly reconfiguring the role of psychiatry today in the broader world of mental health care.

Notes

1. A search of the national press reveals not only frequent articles by Dr Persaud on a range of different topics but also comments by columnists on his ubiquitous presence. For example, see Catherine Bennett in the *Guardian*: 'Should this bright young winner of the Royal College of Psychiatrists' research prize and medal really be squandering quite so much of his talent on Richard and Judy's Good Morning show where he is the "resident psychiatrist"?' (Bennett 2000). In Dr Persaud's defence, he has now ably taken over from Professor Clare on *All in the Mind* on BBC Radio 4 – a programme which encourages debate on mental health issues. Dr Persaud's web page can be located at: www.btinternet.com/~rajendra/

2. In a Balint group, (named after Michael Balint, a psychoanalyst who pioneered the technique with general practitioners), the doctor reflects both on his patient's story and on the impact the patient has on his or her own thoughts and feelings. Through reflection, doctors can come to understand the central importance of the doctor–patient relationship as a therapeutic tool. See Balint (1964).

3. The Care Programme Approach (Department of Health 1990) was a system of co-ordinating care introduced in the UK in an attempt to improve liaison between services in the aftermath of increased concern about risk posed by people with mental health problems living in the community during the 1990s (for policy implementation see www.doh.gov.uk/nsf/polbook.htm), although some who work in the mental health services feel this has led to increasing bureaucracy and paper-chasing without any proven impact on quality of care (Szmukler 2000). The Supervision Register is a locally held list of people who pose a serious risk to themselves (see 'Lions' Den Directive', note 7).

4. Psychiatrists working in the UK National Health Service are paid according to the terms and conditions and salary scales common to all doctors in the NHS (for up-to-date information see www.bmjcareers.com/cgi-bin/section.pl?sn=salary or the inside front page of the careers section in the *British Medical Journal*). However, the shortage of consultants in the last decade has led to some consultants successfully negotiating very generous salary packages above the national pay-scales. A new consultant contract has recently been agreed which will increase salaries. Locum consultants and those working wholly in the private sector negotiate separately.

5. The role of the Responsible Medical Officer (RMO) is only enshrined in UK law in the Mental Health Act (1983) in respect of patients receiving compulsory treatment. According to the Royal College of Psychiatrists (1996), the medical care of outpatients remains 'the ongoing responsibility of general practitioners, with consultants acting in an advisory capacity or providing specialist treatment' (1996: 10). However, 'consultant psychiatrists retain the ultimate responsibility for all aspects of medical care of an in-patient under their care, including discharge' (1996: 10). In the multi-disciplinary team the medical role is 'primary in the process of assessment and/or diagnosis and issues of confidentiality' (1996: 17), and 'consultant psychiatrists can only accept responsibility for a patient of whom they have specific knowledge' (1996: 9). As Kennedy and Griffiths (2002: 205) point out, college statements and other guidance from the General Medical Council do not answer the questions:

(a) To what extent, if any, is the consultant in a multidisciplinary community mental health team (CMHT) responsible for patients being cared for by other secondary care professionals, whom he/she has never seen or whose care he/she is not routinely supervising?

(b) What is, and what is not, medical diagnosis, treatment and care, as distinct from other forms of assessment, therapy or care?

6. **Managed behavioural healthcare organizations** were introduced in an attempt to cut costs, and one of the ways they have done this has been to replace psychiatrists as providers of psychotherapy with much less expensive social workers, psychologists and nurses.

7. In his book, Peter Bruggen (1997) refers to the 'Lions' Den Directive' as the policy that came into being as a result of a chronically psychotic person failing to keep up with his medication and walking into the lions' den at London Zoo – which resulted in headlines in national newspapers. 'James saw the 'lions' den directive – to create a list of people at risk – as little more than a cynical management manoeuvre to show that something had been done: and to create a queue of ready scapegoats' (1997: 165), referring to mental health staff – overstretched and under-resourced – who will be called into account at an inquiry following an 'incident'.

8. Duncan Double manages the Critical Psychiatry Website which contains links to a number of organizations and publications. See http://www.uea.ac.uk/~wp276/psychiatryanti.htm

9. Robert and Françoise Castel developed the term 'psychiatric society' to characterize the alleged domination of twentieth-century western politics by the rationales of the 'psy-complex', which can be seen as a hegemonic value system equivalent to a new religion. See Castel et al. (1982).

10. The caseload of consultant psychiatrists varies considerably, but a general psychiatrist consultant working in a traditional way may have overall responsibility for a large number of outpatients (in the low hundreds) who are only seen intermittently, and a smaller number who are seen more frequently. Once a patient is admitted to hospital (again numbers of available beds may vary considerably – but between ten and fifteen is not unusual) he or she may not be seen as regularly, as day-to-day care is provided by junior doctors. Alternatives to hospitalization, such as day hospital or home treatment services, will be run by a team of mental health workers that includes a psychiatrist.

4

THE SCOPE AND LIMITS OF PSYCHIATRY

Different views prevail in the literature about what is the legitimate business of the psychiatrist. In a recent article in the *British Medical Journal*, Duncan Double (2002), who is active in the Critical Psychiatry Network (see p. 98, note 8) questioned the expansion of psychiatry over recent decades and the process by which common emotional problems have become medicalized. In his view mental health care has come to function as a panacea for many different personal and social problems. He considers that the expansion of psychiatry is reflected in the dramatic increase in the diagnosis of 'attention-deficit disorder' in children for which the prescription of stimulant drugs has considerably increased. But does this necessarily mean that the role of psychiatrists themselves has expanded? While it would be difficult to argue that decisions about psychotropic drug treatment in children are not a responsibility of the child psychiatrist, the major marketing targets of pharmaceutical companies for drugs that treat anxiety and depression are not the psychiatrists but the (much more numerous in our society) general practitioners. Indeed, another view of psychiatry is that its business is contracting back into the role defined in the days of alienism, the care of the 'mad', with possible consequences that include a loss of skills within psychiatry, and increasing demoralization in the profession (Wessely 1996).

In this chapter we will consider what lies within the remit of the profession of psychiatry – exploring the limits of that work and the problems faced in defining where the boundaries lie.

Do psychiatrists only treat 'mental illness'?

Most psychiatrists today would undoubtedly see their major role as treating people who have mental illness. The proportion of these people in the community whom they personally treat (or who are referred to mental health services at all) is in fact quite small, with the large majority being cared for by a range of other professionals in general medical settings and voluntary agencies in the community. The direct involvement of psychiatrists in the management of patients in primary care, the majority of whom suffer from anxiety, depression and adjustment disorders, is highly variable. In the past, psychiatry played a larger part in the management of people with learning disability than they do today. They are now only peripherally involved with this group, carving out a role in the treatment of the mental illness to which people with a learning disability have an excessive liability (Turner 1989).

A problem comes in the management of people whom psychiatrists would, at one extreme of behaviour, diagnose as having a personality disorder, or at the very least a degree of abnormal psychological functioning, or a level of symptomatology that cannot be defined as a psychiatric 'illness'. People with personality difficulties are common in the community and frequently present to general practitioners asking for help with their problems and difficulties in life, many of which are associated with relationships. Many other people may have sexual difficulties, marital problems and complex social difficulties but do not necessarily have the 'disturbance of psychological function' that Lewis (1955) insisted was necessary for a diagnosis of mental illness, although they undoubtedly have a serious disturbance of social functioning. Psychiatrists generally approach this problem in different ways. Anthony Clare comments that:

> Doctors in general medicine ... do not confine themselves to the physically ill either: the pregnant woman, the woman in labour, the person undergoing an examination for a life-assurance policy, the airline pilot having his yearly check-ups, are not necessarily suffering from physical illness yet are properly considered as falling within the physician's area of interest and competence. (Clare 1980: 21)

But, as my colleague Max Marshall, Professor of Community Psychiatry at Manchester University commented to me, psychiatry is 'moving away from treating people for what is presumed to be disease to accepting that we should treat extremes of normal behaviour (such as psychopathy or hyperactivity), 'we are forced to treat society's problems – except you can't treat all society's problems' (interviewed 2003).

Psychiatrists who work closely with those in primary and general medical settings (see below) are much more likely to get involved in providing advice for patients that their colleagues may have decided show 'no evidence of mental illness'. Where clinical psychology services are easily accessible by primary care, they may, however, provide first-line mental health care and advice for this group of people. Both psychiatrists and psychologists are increasingly involved in the assessment of people with serious personality disorders whose anti-social acts and potential dangerousness may have judicial consequences.

Psychiatry and medicine

As Leon Eisenberg remarked, psychiatrists like to think of themselves as the only truly holistic medical speciality. But the truth is that this has occurred rather more by accident than by design:

> Psychiatry made a virtue of the failure of biomedical science to discover effective means for the diagnosis and treatment of psychiatric disorders. If internists learned to focus on organic pathophysiology because it provided the basis for designing specific remedies, we psychiatrists continued to listen to our patients and to study their social interactions, because that alone enabled us to diminish suffering. The ideologies of both specialties have been determined pragmatically. (Eisenberg 1986: 499)

Eisenberg goes on to point out that with the advances in neuroscience, psychiatry may be in danger of falling into the same trap of 'reification of disease that has characterized the other medical specialties' (ibid.: 499). With the developments in neuropsychiatry that are now taking place it is easy to see how this could occur. We will return to considering this in the last chapter of this book, where we look at the future of psychiatry. The question that I want to consider here, however, is where we draw the line between psychiatry and medicine.

It was only during the twentieth century that neurology and psychiatry separated as medical specialities in most countries in the western world, and current advances in neuropsychiatric research make it increasingly difficult to know precisely where to draw the line between neurological and psychiatric disorders (Baker et al. 2002). For example, many patients with Parkinson's disease and stroke manifest depression and, in some cases, dementia. Whatever the views of those who remain antagonistic to biological psychiatry, there is no doubt that the new technologies of functional magnetic resonance imaging (fMRI) and positron emission tomography (PET), together with extensive genetic research, suggest that schizophrenia really is a disorder of the brain. Yet a 'wall' still exists between neurology and psychiatry, as it does between psychiatry and the other medical specialities. Unlike other mental health specialists, psychiatrists are first and foremost trained as doctors and it is this medical knowledge that sets them apart from the other members of the team. However, it could equally be argued that it is the biopsychosocial orientation of psychiatry that truly sets it apart from the rest of medicine. Neurology has traditionally been much more concerned with the complex art of diagnosing rare disorders than with managing the equally complex psychosocial problems faced by people suffering from those rare and incurable neurological disorders. Socially orientated psychiatrists see this as the major reason why neurology will never usurp psychiatry in caring for the mentally ill, even if it becomes 'neuropsychiatry'.

The role of liaison psychiatry

Liaison psychiatry is a speciality that occupies the difficult border-land between psychiatry and medicine, and is sometimes known as 'consultation-liaison psychiatry'. It is primarily concerned with the detection and treatment of psychiatric disorder within the general hospital setting. However, as Richard Mayou (1997) points out, it has two distinct features: it is 'geographical' in that it is specifically concerned with what goes on within the boundaries of the general hospital, and it requires special clinical expertise. The core business of liaison psychiatry is with people who deliberately self-harm and present to general medical services, people with acute behavioural disturbance, patients with **comorbid** physical and psychiatric illness, and those with medically unexplained symptoms, most commonly pain. More specifically, in seeking to treat patients with pain for which no organic lesion can be discovered, liaison psychiatrists challenge the Cartesian, dualistic biomedical model with its focus on the existence of tissue damage in order to explain symptoms.

However, consultation-liaison psychiatry has struggled to achieve recognition within both psychiatry and medicine. One possible reason why it has received little support from fellow psychiatrists is an assumption that consultation-liaison threatens scarce resources for major psychiatric disorders seen in more traditional psychiatric settings (Kessel 1996). Others have suggested this may reflect a wider argument about the scope of psychiatry, as psychiatrists become increasingly preoccupied with traditional mental illness (Wessely 1996), thus reinforcing rather than challenging the dualist split. However, this retreat by psychiatrists into traditional mental illness tends not only to be at the expense of that part of psychiatry allied to medicine, but also to represent a move away from non-psychotic disorders in general in the UK, as government policy has favoured psychiatric resources focusing on 'severe and enduring mental illness'. Nevertheless, in the UK, the reorganization of mental health care into large mental health trusts challenges the integrative ties that psychiatry has built up with general medicine since the opening of the first district general hospital (DGH) mental health units in the mid-twentieth century (Kennedy 2000). Perhaps the next step will be a re-merging of the smaller mental health units into larger mental hospitals. This possibility is already being considered in some places because of the high cost of staffing and running the local mental health units attached to district general hospital units that have been built over the last twenty five years.

Tom Brown is a consultant-liaison psychiatrist who works in Glasgow, and with whom I trained at medical school. He agrees that liaison psychiatrists do not see themselves as particularly favoured by psychiatrists in general. There are far more psychiatrists working in this speciality in North America and Europe, particularly in Holland. He told me:

> Liaison psychiatrists are more esteemed by physicians than they are by their fellow psychiatrists. I've had an almost universally positive experience of colleagues in general hospital, but that may reflect the fact that I have liked working there. In my last job I worked in a general hospital where there was a psychiatric unit within the hospital and in thirteen years I only heard one consultant make a disparaging remark about the presence of the psychiatric unit within the general hospital. General hospital doctors are welcoming of psychiatrists who want to get in there and deal with the kind of things that they see as problems. They are derisory about psychiatrists who see some of the things that trouble them as none of psychiatry's business. (Interviewed 2003)

We discussed the common problem of the patient who deliberately harms himself by cutting his wrist or taking an overdose and regularly turns up at the accident and emergency department, but is shunned by the psychiatric service. Tom Brown said that 'the average general hospital doctor thinks that these patients are very badly dealt with by psychiatrists and doctors are fed up getting letters saying that their patients have a personality disorder and nothing can be done for them – even worse, that they've got no mental illness.' Liaison psychiatrists have expertise in working alongside general medical services to devise management strategies for difficult patients. Like many of his colleagues, Tom thinks that liaison psychiatrists should actually be employed not by mental health trusts but directly by the acute hospital services. However, the reality for liaison psychiatry in the UK has been of a speciality caught at the interface between psychiatry and medicine; moreover, many general hospitals still do not have a consultant-led service, although some clinical psychologists do provide input to specific medical specialities such as neurology.

The *geographical* characteristic of liaison psychiatry delineated by Mayou (1997), in that it is circumscribed by the boundary of the general hospital, can be seen as a weakness rather than a strength. As Tom Brown says:

> There is a bit of a debate, I think, within liaison psychiatry about whether the skills acquired in the pursuit of this kind of territory in a general hospital should not be extended and liaison psychiatrists shouldn't work

with GPs ... If you go to any gathering of liaison psychiatrists they will without a doubt claim expertise in that kind of terrain – what we used to call somatization – and comorbidity with physical illness, and they are somewhat derisory about the average general psychiatrist's ability, but when asked to muck in and take on a bit more they suddenly start to backtrack. (Interviewed 2003)

No doubt this is because liaison psychiatrists are short in numbers, but the history of psychiatry has been to identify itself with institutions, first with the asylum and later, at the start of community psychiatry, with the general hospital. In the United Kingdom, patients now spend much less time in hospital beds, the majority of their physical and emotional care being provided by general practitioners, who have a significant role in planning and commissioning mental health care in the UK.

Psychiatry and family medicine

In countries such as the UK, the Netherlands and Denmark, where primary care physicians act as 'gatekeepers' to specialist services, people with mental health problems have to first consult their primary care physician, also known as family physician or general practitioner, in order to obtain a referral to specialist mental health services. In the UK, such access has been restricted over the last decade as specialist mental health workers, particularly psychiatrists, have limited their remit to working with people who have 'severe and enduring mental illness', usually still defined by diagnosis rather than by limitation of function and taken to be, in practice, schizophrenia, organic mental illness and bipolar disorder. There is an expectation that primary care will increasingly care for the majority of people with mental health problems (Goldberg and Gournay 1997). In the final chapter we will consider the further implications of this policy for *psychiatric practice*.

Ostensibly, psychiatrists should have much in common with general practitioners, or family physicians as they are known in the USA, but their relationship has at times been problematic. Psychotherapeutically orientated psychiatrists have forged relationships with general practitioners, particularly in Europe, over the last half century, beginning with the seminal work of Michael Balint, who brought a psychoanalytic understanding to the relationship between the general practitioner and the patient, and helped doctors reflect on the power of their personal relationship with the patient (Balint 1964; Gask and McGrath 1989).

Across the world, primary care physicians see and treat the majority of people in the community with mental health problems. However, in the UK only about 50 per cent of GPs currently do any psychiatry (normally six months) during their vocational training and this may not prepare them for the mental health problems they commonly see in primary care. GPs expect mental health services therefore to be easily accessible. Wright (1997) has outlined the problems that GPs in the UK perceive with services. They include the geographical remoteness of mental hospitals, poor communication, lack of clarity about management, long waiting lists, problems with urgent referrals, too little contact with mental health professionals, and too few patients being discharged back to general practice care. The UK has a particular tradition of psychiatrists and general practitioners working together. By the 1980s, one-fifth of all general psychiatrists in England and Wales (Strathdee and Williams 1984) and a half in Scotland (Pullen and Yellowlees 1988) were spending some proportion of their time working in primary care. However, a large number of psychiatrists do not spend time in close proximity with primary care, preferring instead to work within the specialist clinic.

In a study that I carried out in a **health maintenance organization** in the USA (Gask, in preparation), I tried to find out why an integrated model of mental health working, which specifically attempted to get psychiatrists, other mental health workers and primary care physicians to work more closely together, had been difficult to roll out to the organization at large, even though it has been demonstrated to be an effective model of working in terms of improved patient outcomes for people suffering from depression (see Katon et al. 1996). Cost was clearly a barrier (integrated care cost more than routine care) even though it was more effective. However, covert attitudinal differences between psychiatrists, other mental health therapists and primary care physicians were also important in preventing integration from reaching the top of the 'change' agenda.

The way in which many mental health professionals work, eschewing interruption and still maintaining the psychoanalytic tradition of the 'fifty-minute hour' even today, militates against fast access to specialists:

> We had a therapist here that was on call one night and a Physician's Assistant who gets more awards than anyone else in this clinic knocked on her door and she said go away don't bother me I'm with a patient. We can't do that. I think you just poison your relationships. (Psychiatrist)

> It requires I think a kind of flexibility that a lot of practitioners in our field don't have. I think many people want to sit in their office and see people on the hour and go home. (Psychologist)

Two conceptual differences between primary care physicians and mental health care specialists in how they view their roles in helping people with problems were identified. First, there was a tension between the 'medical' model of distress shared by most of the primary care physicians (though certainly not all) and the psychiatrists, particularly when it came to managing people with moderately severe mental health problems, and the 'personal responsibility model' favoured by non-medical therapists and other primary care physicians:

> The medical staff say, 'I'm the doctor, I'm calling and I want this person seen, see him.' You know the therapists take more of a stance that it's their [the patient's] responsibility. If they want it, they need to want to come. (Mental health service manager)

This tension bubbled under the surface not just between primary care and mental health but also between the mental health professionals – between the psychiatrists and the Master's level therapists (usually with a social work background). There was, in addition, the mutual misunderstanding about the nature of primary and specialist care. Primary care has little time to pay attention to detail, because, unlike specialist care, it has highly permeable boundaries and easy access for patients:

> Ask a psychiatrist if they're going to have same-day access ... Of course they're not, that's not going to work ... but we're taking care of all-comers wherever they are .... (Primary care physician)

> Someone comes in having dizzy spells and lightheadedness, and this horrible back pain, and also 'my marriage is breaking up and I'm depressed and I'm seeing spots and my left eye went blind yesterday for fifteen minutes, does that mean anything doctor?' (Primary care physician)

The expertise of the primary care physician is in managing the *breadth* of problems. He or she is a 'specialist generalist'. A mental health worker expressed exasperation that his special expertise in understanding human relationships in *depth* was not valued by primary care staff:

> You're around people who are talking about the human condition and its psychological implications and your conversations are in detail about the intricacies of people's lives ... then you walk into a primary care setting where that kind of information really isn't valued very much and they really don't want to know it, they haven't got the time to listen to it. (Social worker)

And indeed many primary care physicians are simply not sufficiently interested in mental health issues to want to know about the detail.

They may be far more enthusiastic about treating one or more of the other problems that health policy dictates they are 'ideally placed' to manage, such as diabetes or cardiovascular disease. The problem, however, is that people with mental health problems may not be able to access help except through or from their primary care physicians, which may to the patient seem highly unsatisfactory, as we found in a study of patients' views of care that they received for depression in primary care. One patient recounted a conversation with her GP:

> I said to him 'look I need help, you'll have to get me to see a psychologist or a psychiatrist' – 'Oh there's a big waiting list you'll have to wait so many months.' And I just thought well this is waste. I had nowhere to turn to.' (Gask et al. 2003: 280)

Current advice about which of their patients general practitioners should refer to mental health services as printed in the *World Health Organization Guide to Common Mental Disorders and Emotional Problems* can be found in Box 5. In the UK most general practitioners are able

---

Box 5   Advice on when to refer a person for a mental health assessment (from WHO 2000).

1. The patient is displaying signs of suicidal intent or if there seems to be a risk of harm to others.
2. The patient is so disabled by their mental disorder that they are unable to leave their home, look after their children or fulfil other activities of daily living.
3. The GP requires the expertise of secondary care to confirm a diagnosis or implement specialist treatment.
4. The GP feels that the therapeutic relationship with the patient has broken down, primary-care interventions and voluntary/non-statutory options have been exhausted.
5. There is severe physical deterioration of the patient.
6. Particular psychotropic medication is required, e.g. clozapine.
7. If the patient requests a referral.

---

only to refer to the 'mental health team' without being able to specify which professional he or she would like to be involved. This decision is made by the mental health team. The extent of involvement of psychiatrists in such teams varies considerably according to levels of staffing and personal style of working, but individuals who have psychotic symptoms and/or are considered to be at highest 'risk' (discussed further below) will usually be seen by the psychiatrist. A minority of psychiatrists, as indicated above, will conduct their clinics in the setting of family practice. Finally, an even smaller number will work much more closely with the family doctor, regularly meeting to discuss patients about whom the doctor wants some advice – a practice known as 'consultation-liaison' (similar to consultation-liaison working in the general hospital setting – see Gask et al. 1997).

Psychiatry: self, state and culture

The history of what constitutes *psychiatric disorder* is, as we have seen, fraught with disagreement and controversy. The psychoanalytic influence on psychiatry probably served, more than any other factor in the last century, to broaden the remit of what might be considered to be of interest to the psychiatrist in the human psyche.

The politics of diagnosis and treatment

It is only relatively recently that homosexuality was determined to be no longer a psychiatric disorder (Bayer 1981), which undoubtedly reflects changes in society and the political success of the gay movement rather than any scientific development in the psychiatric literature (Mechanic 1999b). In his fascinating book *Rewriting the Soul: Multiple Personality and the Science of Memory* (1995), Ian Hacking, a philosopher, drawing on Foucault's concept of the archaeology of knowledge (Foucault 1972), explores how beliefs about multiple personality, always a controversial diagnosis in psychiatry, have developed over the last hundred years. Hacking shows how ideas about the diagnosis and aetiology of multiple personality disorder have changed over time and how it has now come to be linked with ideas about early childhood sexual abuse and the phenomenon of 'recovered' memories, another highly controversial issue which elicits strong opposing feelings and views. Not only does this demonstrate how one branch of psychiatry (mostly in North America) has popularized the diagnosis, but 'did not discover that early and repeated child abuse causes multiple personality; it forged that connection, in the way that a blacksmith turns formless molten metal into tempered steel' (Hacking 1995: 94).

Multiple personality disorder has become a psychological issue in its own right and Hacking rightly asks about the political issues this creates for the US system of health care where insurers prefer drug treatment to psychotherapy:

Who will finally own the illness: highly qualified clinicians with years of training or a populist alliance of patients and therapists who welcome a culture of multiples and who cultivate personalities? ... Dissociation doctors must capture as much non-drug coverage for dissociative disorders as they can ... That will be a top item on the agenda for the medical wing of multiple personality. (Hacking 1995: 53)

Similar political discussions about the nature of diagnosis, have, almost in reverse, occurred with the discussion about the nature of chronic fatigue syndrome, (popularly known as 'ME'). Despite arguments to the contrary by leading psychiatrists that it may respond to psychological treatments, the UK Department of Health has announced that it is *not* a 'mental' problem. This has partly come about in response to a powerful lobby of sufferers who find the psychological explanation demeaning and disempowering, but it also raises the question, asked by Hacking, about who owns a diagnosis and who is the 'expert'.

The expert patient: post-modernism and psychiatry

Most of us will be familiar with the following situation. We have seen and assessed a patient and have given advice as to the most appropriate management. The person listens attentively then says he or she does not agree with the proposed treatment and feels an alternative would be more suited to his or her needs. The psychiatrist explains that according to the available evidence, the suggested management is the most effective and the alternative, which might be very expensive in cost, does not usually work for the patient's problem. The patient replies that what works for the majority would not necessarily work for them, and that he or she feels confident about knowing what will be effective. (Laugharne 1999: 641)

In his paper 'Evidence-based medicine, user involvement and the post-modern paradigm' Richard Laugharne (1999) points to the conflict faced by the practising psychiatrist who is encouraged to use the 'modernist' paradigm of 'evidence-based medicine' (see Chapter 2) in a post-modern world which no longer holds to objective reality, but to the relative reality for that individual participating in the process. The central values of post-modern theory, although it is notoriously difficult to define, seem to be those of uncertainty, difference in views and experiences of reality, and multi-faceted descriptions of 'truth'.

Arthur W. Frank argues that 'postmodern experience of illness begins when ill people recognize that more is involved in their experiences than the medical story can tell' (1996: 6). We can see the consumer or user movement, as it is called in mental health contexts, and the move towards 'patient-centred' medicine that has been powerful in family practice as reflections of the increasing acknowledgement of post-modern trends in health care. Some aspects of current health policy in the west support the view that, particularly in chronic illness, the patient is the 'expert' in his or her own symptoms and illness experience. However, this does not sit easily with the constant exhortations faced by the clinician at the front-line to use 'evidence-based medicine'. A good example of how these two approaches may be at odds can be seen in the recent publication of two reports from a piece of work commissioned by the UK Department of Health. The systematic review of randomized controlled trials published recently in the *Lancet* conducted by John Geddes and colleagues in the UK ECT Review Group (2003) concluded that 'ECT is an effective short-term treatment for depression, and is probably more effective than drug therapy.' They limited their discussion to interpretation of the science without consideration of the acceptability of ECT as a treatment in practice. Rose and her colleagues (2003) three months later published a systematic review of patients' perspectives on ECT and stated that 'although clinical trials concluded that electroconvulsive therapy is an effective treatment, measures of efficacy did not take into account all the factors that may lead patients to perceive it as beneficial or otherwise'.

Politicians meanwhile feel able to pursue the 'evidence-based' trajectory and support the concept of the 'expert patient' without acknowledging how this potentially problematizes the negotiations of diagnosis and treatment between patient and professional. Nowhere is this currently more evident than in the field of psychiatric care in the UK where a political agenda of increasing coercion is being pursued (see p. 123).

Psychiatry and politics
Psychiatric diagnosis has always been inexorably liked with politics but perhaps never as overtly as in the abuse of psychiatry that took place in the Soviet Union and is alleged to be currently taking place in China.

> In the former Soviet Union during the Krushchev–Breznev era, the KGB used its forensic psychiatric institutions to brand, arbitrarily and for political reason, large numbers of political dissidents as suffering from 'schizophrenia' and 'paranoid psychosis' and then incarcerated them for long periods in 'special psychiatric hospitals'. In 1976, the Soviet Union was severely censured on this account by psychiatrists from all over the world at a conference in Hawaii of the World Psychiatric Association. Only after Gorbachev's rise to power were these errors rectified. We have now discovered that similar practices have also occurred in parts of China. (Jia Yicheng, China's top forensic psychiatrist in 1998, quoted in Munro 2002: 1)

In 1987 it was estimated that of 800 well-documented cases of political prisoners in the USSR, 20 per cent were hospitalized (Finlayson 1987). Anatoly Koryagin, who had been psychiatric adviser to the Moscow Committee monitoring the Helsinki Accord on Human Rights, examined sixteen dissenters who had either been in a mental hospital or were at risk of being sent there because of their political beliefs. He spent six years in a labour camp and internal exile before being released. The majority of Soviet psychiatrists undoubtedly quietly acquiesced, but the Soviet Psychiatric Association, facing almost certain expulsion, voluntarily withdrew from the WPA in 1983 and was readmitted after the Gorbachev reforms led to the release of most psychiatrically detained critics of the regime. The Soviet Union was, however, not alone in detaining political dissidents in mental hospital and the People's Republic of China also detained large numbers of dissidents in this way. Recently, there has been criticism of China's treatment of members of the Falun Gong movement (a meditative movement drawing on several Eastern religious doctrines). Munro estimates that at least 600 practitioners of Falun Gong have been forcibly assigned psychiatric treatment in an attempt to compel them to renounce their beliefs. At the WPA Congress in Yokohama in 2002 there was extensive debate and pressure on the WPA from some speakers, particularly those involved in the Geneva Initiative on Psychiatry[1] to expel the Chinese association, although this has so far resulted only in an agreement to conduct an independent international inquiry (Lyons and O'Malley 2002; van Voren 2002). Meanwhile, another commentator suggested that, while we should deplore the situation in China, we must not be complacent about the rights and treatment of the mentally ill at home:

> I always felt a strong sense of irony and shame chairing meetings of the Ethics Sub-committee, where unethical behaviour overseas was regularly subjected to critical scrutiny in the comfortable surrounding of Belgrave Square, only to return to my own practice in East London, where patients (many of them compulsorily detained and lacking any sort of choice) often had to sleep on floors, in dilapidated acute admission wards with little possibility of access to psychological therapies, decent occupational therapy or any adequate provision for care in the community. (Deahl 2002: 446)

In order to address these problems, some psychiatrists feel they have no option but to become politically active in the broadest sense, either through the Royal College or, more radically, by arguing that psychiatry, as a profession, has failed (Bracken and Thomas 2001).

Recognizing the importance of values

Evaluations of the presence or absence of a 'psychiatric disorder' are, as we have seen, made by systematic assessment of a person's mental state and the history of their problems, as reported by the person themselves and significant others or 'informants'. However, it becomes clearer that what is often not adequately addressed is that the values of the observer, professional or non-professional, will influence these judgements and will depend on the cultural, social, religious and political context in which people live and work.

Psychiatrists conventionally divide mental disorder into three categories: mental illness, severe learning disability and personality disorder. What constitutes an 'illness' or 'disease' is not quite so clear, however, and the principal model of disease in psychiatry, despite the technical advances of the twentieth century in understanding abnormalities of brain structure and functioning, remains the syndrome model. A syndrome is an identifiable cluster of symptoms and signs which are associated with a characteristic course over time but without a clearly determined pathological process identified. In other medical specialities, where the pathological determinants of the disease can be identified, the 'syndrome' model has been superseded by the 'disease' model.[2] However, it is easy to see why the disease model is so attractive to psychiatrists. If an underlying brain abnormality (or abnormalities) can be identified, as is becoming apparent in schizophrenia, there is a logical case for saying that, as the pattern of symptoms which constitutes schizophrenia is a syndrome recognized across the world in many different cultures, then this must be a 'real' mental illness, with an underlying identifiable (if not yet fully identified) disease process, which falls firmly within the remit of the psychiatrist.

The apparent simplicity of this argument, supported as it is by the wealth of neuropsychiatric research of the last twenty years (Andreasen 2001) demonstrating that there are indeed biological changes in the brains of people to whom psychiatrists would give a diagnosis of schizophrenia, belies the complex social and political tapestry within which the clinical psychiatrist has to function in order to diagnose accurately and treat people whom he would recognize as suffering from schizophrenia or any other mental disorder.

Culture and ethnicity

Psychiatric researchers have determined that although syndromes such as schizophrenia can be recognized universally by researchers across cultures,[3] they are not universally recognized by health workers as 'illness' and therefore treated. Western psychiatrists promote recognition of depression as important across all cultures, through the work of organizations such as the WPA and WHO, but the way in which people present as 'depressed', and the values attached by society to those symptoms, vary considerably across the world. To deal with these variations, clinical psychiatrists must make a distinction between the 'essential pathogenic determinants of a mental disorder, those biological processes which are held to be necessary and sufficient to cause it, and the **pathoplastic** personal and cultural variations in the pattern' (Littlewood 1996).[4] Arthur Kleinman's fascinating ethnographic studies of the practice of psychiatry in both North America and China further reveal the way in which the psychiatrist's 'experience of the self, his intuitive grasp of the dynamics of other selves and his clinical work ... arise from an interplay of these universal and culturally particular elements in psychology' (Kleinman 1991: 99). Kleinman asserts that 'an anthropological sensibility regarding the cultural uses and social uses of the diagnostic process can be an effective check on its potential misuses and abuses' (ibid.: 17). Suman Fernando, a British psychiatrist, takes these ideas further, challenging the implicit and overt racism within European psychiatry (Fernando 1988).

The ability to practise a 'culturally sensitive' psychiatry, as espoused by Kleinman and Fernando, is as essential to psychiatrists working in their own countries and, ostensibly, familiar cultures, as it is to those who train in the west and seek to return to improve the provision of services in developing countries. Commenting on Littlewood (1996), Bhugra and Cochrane argue that:

> Health professionals often tend to treat culture as an ambiguous concept belonging to 'other' rather than themselves. They may deprecate culture as something secondary to biological models within the biopsychosocial approaches to diagnosis and management of psychiatric disorders. (Bhugra and Cochrane 2001: 18)

Psychiatrists often face considerable criticism about the overrepresentation of people from certain ethnic minority groups among those detained in hospital and/or given a diagnosis of schizophrenia in the UK (Bhugra and Cochrane 2001). The terminology used for this branch of psychiatry is open to critical debate.

Dinesh Bhugra, Dean of the Royal College of Psychiatrists and a consultant in South London told me:

> My personal preference is cultural psychiatry, because one of the problems of transcultural psychiatry has been that it is always seen as ex-colonial masters looking at ex-colonial populations – whether they are migrants or not. The way in which psychiatrists (in the UK) started off

looking at ethnic minorities was slightly esoteric. In the fifties and the sixties there were two schools of thought. One was that these poor people needed to be protected from themselves and therefore people went in with very medical models saying they're 'all ill' or 'not ill at all'. The second one was a very kind of Marxist ideological model, that because ethnic minorities had been imported into this country as cheap labour the capitalist model of production controlled what was being done and said ... Within that, health didn't arise as an issue. Then there was a very liberal phase and people started flying the flag that schizophrenia had been overdiagnosed, almost a Laingian perspective that society was creating illness. In the last fifteen years or so the pendulum has swung again to a more reasoned debate, but still irrational I think, about whether certain disorders are more frequent or not and what are the possible explanations.

In some countries, such as the USA and Canada in particular, there has been a clear move among researchers in cultural psychiatry away from looking at migrant populations and towards the needs of the indigenous populations. Dinesh Bhugra is in no doubt that incidence rates among African Caribbeans for schizophrenia are higher than in the white population in the UK, but thinks that the reasons for this are complex. 'If you look at people who are being entered into these studies, it's not the psychiatrists that are diagnosing schizophrenia, it's the families that are diagnosing abnormal behaviour which is bringing them in – they need help.' Psychiatry is often viewed with suspicion by people from ethnic minority populations, partly because of the stigma of mental illness and because they have different models for viewing what would be seen in European culture as a 'mental health problem', but also, according to Dinesh Bhugra,

> it goes back to 'everything is institutionally racist'.... Some of it is a genuine fear, but some of it is exaggerated by various folk because that is their *raison d'être*. For young black men I've seen in the ward, you say 'you need to take this medication', and they say 'you would say that, wouldn't you, you're being paid to control, paid to do this', and no matter how you try ... they are just not interested ... people come in saying quite openly that you are misdiagnosing all these poor black people and that somehow there has been a conspiracy. To me that feels that there is a massive degree of distrust.

Elaine Arnold, who specializes in psychiatry of the elderly, succinctly summarized for me the political and cultural issues inherent in making a diagnosis:

> If I say there is a higher incidence of multi-infarct dementia in Afro-Caribbean males because of a higher incidence of malignant hypertension – that is seen as a value-free statement. But if you say there is a

higher incidence of schizophrenia ... that is a whole different thing altogether. (Interviewed 2003)

So it is difficult to consider issues of race and culture without also considering the influence of politics on the scope and limits of psychiatry.

Psychiatry and the nature of religious experience

The interaction between religion and the practice of psychiatry is also complex. Bhugra (1996, citing Nelson and Torrey 1973) has noted that: 'Increasingly, mental health practitioners are assuming the three functions traditionally associated as being in the domain of religion. First, an explanation of the unknown. Second, ritual and social function, and, third, the definition of values' (Bhugra 1996: 2).

He goes on to describe how the interaction between religion and psychiatry can be at several levels. Psychiatric patients may have certain religious beliefs that need to be taken into account when planning management. They may seek help from religion and religious healers who view the nature and causes of psychological distress quite differently from mental health professionals. In my own experience I can think of patients who have looked for explanations from eastern mysticism or become involved with religious groups, mainstream or marginal, during the period when they were seeking explanations and help for their strange or disturbing experiences. In my attempt to convey the anthropological sensitivity advocated by Kleinman (1991), I have treated my patients with western pharmacology as an adjunct to specific religious remedies prescribed by the Muslim teacher or Imam. I have sought out the hospital chaplain for depressed patients racked with guilt about crimes they have not committed, in the knowledge that, for them, treatment will require, from a representative of God, confession, forgiveness and reassurance that I could not provide.

However, what is often most difficult for psychiatrists in training is coming to terms with the way that symptoms of one kind may be viewed differently by someone else who holds particular religious and/or cultural beliefs. Our patients and/or their families and acquaintances may interpret their symptoms in particular ways. They may believe themselves to be reincarnations of religious figures or hear the voice of God commanding them to carry out tasks. Some of these experiences resonate with the descriptions of the religious experiences of famous saints and mystics. Modern psychiatry defines itself as essentially a 'scientific' discipline and psychiatrists have not restricted themselves to *post-hoc* diagnoses of the madness of kings (see Chapter 1). These psychobiographies of historical figures who have experienced religious visions, trances or other transcendental happenings have tended to biological reductionism (Lipsedge 1996), an activity warned against by the psychologist William James over a century ago in his masterful study of *The Varieties of Religious Experience*:

> Medical materialism seems indeed a good appellation for the too simple-minded system of thought which we are considering. Medical materialism finishes up Saint Paul by calling his vision on the road to Damascus a discharging lesion of the occipital cortex, he being an epileptic. It snuffs out St Teresa as an hysteric ... then thinks that the spiritual authority of all such personages is undermined. (James 1977: 35)

As Bill Fulford, who holds a Chair in both Psychiatry and Philosophy, notes, 'reductionism might seem to offer an attractive philosophical strategy for psychiatry, spanning as it does the mind/ brain divide' (1996: 13). However, he argues that psychiatrists must keep clear sight of the relationship between facts and values as 'twin and equally essential attributes of persons' (ibid.: 16).

Psychiatry in the community

Thus, the role of psychiatry in the broader community is – based on what we have considered so far – open to considerable debate. In his seminal paper 'Who ought to see a psychiatrist?' Neil Kessel (1963) was rightly critical of a profession that he saw, by the mid-twentieth century, to have oversold itself, echoing Aubrey Lewis (1955), who had earlier observed: 'It may be that there is no form of social deviation in an individual which psychiatrists will not claim to treat or prevent – the pretensions of some psychiatrists are extreme.' Media psychiatrists notwithstanding, most psychiatrists today would dissociate themselves from the excesses of the last century when psychiatrists, particularly in North America, fuelled by psychoanalytic insights, offered therapeutic help and interpretations for ills that extended far beyond the remit of what is today recognized, by psychiatrists at least, as 'mental illness'. But where does psychiatry draw the boundary? Even today, when most psychiatrists in the UK limit themselves to the management of 'major' psychiatric illness (schizophrenia, bipolar disorder, organic disorders), they can still be criticized for acting as the policemen of the state in detaining 'deviant' individuals in hospital, demonstrating racism in the rate at which they detain people from ethnic minorities, and committing a range of other potential social crimes in their dealings with those whom they believe to be in need (or definitely not in need) of their help. It is a difficult job to do without offending anyone at all – not only because the boundaries are not clear, but because they are often defined by others, including politicians and, increasingly, the media.

Defining and delivering 'community psychiatry'

Nikolas Rose, commenting on the emergence of community psychiatry, sees this movement as a way for psychiatry to 'modernize' itself and for psychiatrists to 'respond to critiques of their custodial and controlling role by seeking to divest their activities of their anti-liberal and 'carceral' features, sloughing these off to other forms of expertise so that psychiatry can become a liberal, open and curative medicine' (Rose 1996: 5). However, he goes on to add:

> What is of particular interest in the emergence of the rationalities of community psychiatry is the novel role that is accorded to psychiatric experts; less that of curing illness than of *administering pathological individuals across an archipelago of specialist institutions and types of activity*, and simultaneously engaging in a prophylactic and preventative work of maximizing mental health. (ibid.: 5, italics added).

Rose raises important questions about what we actually mean by community care, and questions the nature of the administrative role played by psychiatry.

At a time when the concept of 'care in the community' in the UK has become tarnished with government statements of failure, it can be difficult to remember how and why the idea of community psychiatry first came about. In 1946 Blacker used it to distinguish between a 'closed hospital psychiatry' for mentally retarded and psychotic patients, and psychiatry 'in the outside world', concerned with the treatment of people with neurotic illness (Blacker 1946). However, it came into common usage in Britain in the late 1950s with the development of a policy for treating people without bringing them into hospital or discharging them sooner than had occurred in the past. In the 1960s, the way in which community services developed differed on each side of the Atlantic. In the USA, community mental health centres, which were strongly influenced by the public health model of Caplan (1964), failed in their over-ambitious aim to 'prevent mental illness' in the community. In the UK, community psychiatry came to be used to describe the national plan for mental health services based around new district general hospital psychiatric units with access to an increasing range of specialist services. Later, this would evolve into a model close to that familiar today in UK mental health care, with the development of multi-disciplinary community-based mental health teams serving particular geographically defined 'sectors' of the population. As Bennett and Freeman have commented: 'To be effective such a practice would need to be grounded in social psychiatry, i.e. the relationship of social factors to psychiatric illness and of that illness to society: it involved the aim of caring not just for the identified patient but for a whole population over a significant period of time' (Bennett and Freeman 1991: 2). The extent to which such a community-orientated psychiatric service would differentially benefit a range of people, from those who would formerly have been at risk of becoming long-stay mental patients to those people who might never have even seen a psychiatrist, remains a topic of debate.

I share Max Marshall's views on the demise of the mental hospital. 'Asylums were awful places – people lived miserable lives there.' Max is one of the foremost among the new breed of more specialized community psychiatrists who, in the last fifteen years, have developed a speciality within general psychiatry which focuses on the care of the neediest disabled people with mental illness living in the community. In one sense, all general psychiatrists are now community psychiatrists by default, because the community is where care is provided and where all psychiatrists should be trained to work. Psychiatrists in training require the confidence and experience to be able to carry out assessment and management of problems in the GP's surgery, the patient's home, the police station or on the street if needed, as well as in the familiar security of the hospital setting (Littlejohns et al. 1992). Max is quite sure that the people, whom the **Assertive Community Treatment**, or ACT, team work with, want to live in the community, but this brings its dilemmas for those caring for these patients. 'The new generation wants to be in the community and has to be intensively cared for in the community ... They are more independent and have more means at hand to be self-destructive, yet on the other hand they have much better lives than hospitalized patients did.' A problem faced by most, if not all, psychiatrists trying to develop effective community-based services has been that the resources released when the great mental hospitals were closed, and their prime sites sold off to property developers and supermarkets, did not get channelled back into re-provision of intensive, well-staffed, highly skilled and truly multi-disciplinary community services – which has understandably led to some disillusionment (Robertson 1994). Thornicroft and Goldberg, responding to the question, 'Has community care failed?' concluded that the jury should still be out because community care has only been half-implemented. The complete range of community services advocated by the UK Department of Health is not yet to be found anywhere:

Its implementation has been *half-minded* because our services haven't been based upon even the evidence that we have to hand, and it has been *half-hearted* because we haven't yet had a full commitment to provide services of a standard that all of us would find acceptable if we or our families were treated within them. We owe it to ourselves, to the mentally ill and to their families to do better than this. (Thornicroft and Goldberg 1998: 23)

According to the UK government, the policy of community care has failed, despite evidence to the contrary that adequately funded initiatives can improve the quality of people's lives.[5] Psychiatrists attempting to implement effective systems of care in the community find themselves between a rock and a hard place.

On the one hand there is the rising public alarm at perceived 'random attacks by mentally ill people', fuelled to some degree by the media, and leading to implementation of policy driven by fear. Mental illness has come to be linked in the minds of the public with violence. However, research has consistently failed to establish that the mentally ill are responsible for more than a minority of homicides and indeed are more likely to be victims than perpetrators (Hiroeh et al. 2001). Society in general is becoming more violent and this is reflected in the behaviour of the mentally ill, particular in connection with the increasing use of illicit drugs which fuel a considerable amount of the psychosis seen by psychiatrists who work in inner cities. The UK government has responded to public concern, however, by introducing new and increasingly coercive legislation (see p. 123) and promoting, at least in the view of mental health professionals, an unrealistic vision of a world where risk of such incidents can be minimized to the point of extinction. In the firing line in this new culture, fuelled by fear and blame, are the psychiatrists, who find themselves increasingly subject to inquiries following each incident. Psychiatrists are criticized if they do not ensure that severely ill patients are receiving appropriate care, which inevitably means medication. However, as journalist Jeremy Laurance comments in his study of services for the mentally ill in Britain,

Many psychiatrists take a wider view and would like to attend to other things in patients' lives than medication but they are constrained in reality. The imperative that drives the service is risk avoidance and damage limitation – to lives lived on the edge. What inner city psychiatrists worry about is having to stand up in court to explain their management of a case. When that happens they know they will have to defend themselves in terms of the prevailing view of appropriate treatment – that is drugs. (Laurance 2003: 6)

Treating the patient or protecting the public?

As Adshead (1999: 321) has pointed out, the 'duties of a doctor' according to the UK General Medical Council, are 'generally seen as being owed to a particular patient or patients, and not to the community at large'. Psychiatrists who work with the chronically ill appreciate the importance of relatives and carers, but there are no hard and fast rules, or legal precedents, to dictate how much relatives should be involved. In my practice I have generally tried to involve relatives, with the patient's permission, whenever possible, but I am always careful to respect a patient's wishes for confidentiality. In the event, I have only broken the rule of confidentiality when I have been seriously concerned about the safety of another person, adult or child, and felt that I needed to take steps to ensure their safety, involving where necessary the appropriate authorities such as child-care agencies and the police.

In the Tarasoff case (Tarasoff v. Regents of the University of California et al. 1976), Tatiana Tarasoff was killed by a man who had previously told his therapist of his homicidal thoughts towards Miss Tarasoff. The California Supreme Court ruled that the therapist's duty of care was 'trumped' by the claims of the potential victim. Adshead (1999), summarizing the outcomes of recent high-profile cases in the UK (including the case of Christopher Clunis)[6] and current official guidance for doctors (Department of Health, 1990 and General Medical Council 1995), concludes that:

- Psychiatrists may have a duty to prevent their patients from acting criminally if the patient is so ill that they either (a) do not know what they are doing or (b) do not know that it is wrong.
- Doctors have a duty to breach confidentiality and warn an identifiable victim where there is a possible risk from a patient.

Determining and managing risk

Views about detaining patients for assessment and treatment lie at the heart of the philosophical differences between mental health professionals both in and outside psychiatry. If you view, as most working psychiatrists do, mental illness as something which exists 'out there' and which needs to be detected and treated, then you will find it easier to justify detaining a person for assessment and/or treatment under mental health law. If you do not believe in the concept of 'mental illness' and/or find the idea of treating a person against their will impossible to accept, this will be difficult for you. For many health professionals, including GPs who often find detention of patients they know well very difficult, working in the therapeutic relationship in collaboration with the patient will always be in conflict with any suggestion of treating them against their will. Many psychiatrists will say, and indeed I have experienced this myself, that there are patients who will later thank you for treating them, even though it involved detaining them, because although they did not recognize they needed treatment at the time they came to see this later. Equally, there are patients with whom a relationship built on trust is never possible after you have 'sectioned' them. There is, however, a growing debate in the UK about whether the psychiatrist who is caring for the patient should retain the role of being the person who makes the decision to detain that person (Turner et al. 1999; Bracken and Thomas 2001). A further problem arises when the psychiatrist, as legally responsible medical officer, then retains that responsibility regardless of whether other legal avenues of appeal cause the patient to be discharged into the community.

Generally, when psychiatrists consider detention, it is because the person is considered to be (a) suffering from a mental disorder and (b) considered to be a risk to himself or to others. (The wording and exact remit of mental health law varies across the world, from nation to nation, and even within the British Isles.) Detention allows for assessment and treatment in hospital. Involuntary treatment outside hospital remains controversial among British psychiatrists although it has been implemented in some parts of the world (McIvor 2001).

From a psychiatric point of view, suicide is seen as essentially preventable if the person is suffering from a treatable mental illness such that the suicidal ideation would no longer be expressed if the person received and responded to treatment adequately. Psychiatrists' views of whether a person should be actively prevented from trying to kill himself or herself may differ from those of other health professionals, and from more psychodynamically oriented psychiatrists working primarily as psychotherapists, who do not see their role as making a judgement about a person's right to 'rationally' decide to take their life. As a non-psychiatric mental health professional said about psychiatrists during an interview in a recent research project with which I was personally involved:

> The SHOs [junior doctors] say from time to time our job is to keep people alive, and that reminds me that they're coming from a very different place to me. Not that I don't think it's my job to help people; well, my job isn't to keep people alive – it may be to help people to find reasons for wanting to continue to be alive.

But the job of the psychiatrist not only involves keeping his or her patient alive but also preventing the patient harming others in the community. Castel (1991) has argued that there has recently been a shift from thinking about 'dangerousness' to thinking about 'risk' in mental health policy. Notions of risk management have reshaped the obligations of mental health professionals, particularly psychiatrists.

The logic of predictions comes to replace the logic of diagnosis – and this is a logic in which the psychiatrists can claim no special competence. What is at stake is the classification of the subjects of psychiatry in terms of likely future conduct, their riskiness to the community and themselves and identification of the steps necessary to manage that conduct. And within this rationale, the medical institution is redefined – no longer a place of cure, it becomes little more than a container for the most risky until their riskiness can be fully assessed and controlled. (Rose 1996: 16)

Protecting the public?

So how far does the psychiatrist's duty to protect the public extend? Adshead (1999) points out that the primary aim of existing UK mental health legislation is the protection of the health and well-being of people with mental illnesses. However, the proposed new mental health legislation in England and Wales includes plans for the piloting of a new service for the assessment and treatment of people with 'dangerous severe personality disorder' (DSPD), a diagnosis devised and defined by government rather than by the medical profession, 'under the unashamed banner of public protection' (Chiswick 2001). The same author has also commented that 'the folly of equating high risk with a dubious psychiatric diagnosis to the exclusion of other relevant factors cannot be overemphasized'(Chiswick 1999: 704).

Cawthra and Gibb are clear (as far as this is possible) about the role of psychiatry in the management of severe personality disorder:

Difficult and disturbed individuals within society will continue to present a challenge, but this not does mean that psychiatry should necessarily provide treatment for those that society finds unmanageable and unacceptable by means of their behaviour ... to expect psychiatry to contain those with severe personality disorder for long periods of time when there is no realistic prospect of significant therapeutic benefit seems a misuse of precious hospital resources. (Cawthra and Gibb 1998: 9)

There is additionally concern about both the serious threat to human rights and the demonizing of the mentally ill that such detention poses. Psychiatrists have united with other mental health professionals and users of services and carers to oppose the legislation.

However, Maden warns against psychiatry relying on whether something is 'treatable' to define its boundaries of responsibility:

The refusal to help patients who are acknowledged to have a disease, just because they are unlikely to get better, violates all of medicine's ethical principles. It is also bad science in that medical progress would be impossible if doctors washed their hands of every disease for which treatment is uncertain. The damage caused by this attitude should not be underestimated. There are few more depressing sights than the complacency with which some psychiatrists will diagnose an untreatable personality disorder, conclude that supervision is impossible – then leave a probation officer to carry out the supervision. (Maden 1999: 708)

My colleague, Jenny Shaw, who is a Senior Lecturer in Forensic Psychiatry at the University of Manchester, has some sympathies with this view:

Traditionally the treatment of personality disorder in this country has been the domain of psychologists, certainly in secure settings, and I think there has been a lot of woolly thinking among psychiatrists with some saying it's not treatable at all. … Other psychiatrists go to the other extreme and will discuss treatability … . I think psychiatrists haven't got their act together over personality disorder and in secure settings psychologists have come in and tried to establish some parameters of working with these people. (Interviewed 2003)

But neither personality disorder nor dangerousness constitute 'disease' as a physician would recognize it, although they may be markers of a 'diseased society'. Maden does not support the detention of people in hospital on the grounds of personality disorder alone, but supports the development and testing of a range of therapeutic interventions aimed at addressing personality disorder. The medium secure units in the NHS are already under pressure to take more and more mentally ill people out of prison and detention of more people with a diagnosis of personality disorder will potentially further increase this load. To some of us, the NHS secure units seem like a new version of an old and familiar institution in psychiatry, the asylum. As Jenny Shaw said to me:

I work at the site of an old asylum. I too have looked back at the history of it and it's very interesting because we are sort of re-inventing it now but with locked doors, I suppose. The site where I worked used to have industrial therapy, a farm, and with our new, growing, long-stay population we are looking at re-inventing a farm for example and industrial-type occupations. (Interviewed 2003)

Could this be yet another case of 'back to the future' as society re-invents the self-sufficient asylum? We will consider the possible futures that notable experts have predicted for psychiatry in the last chapter.

Notes

1. The Geneva Initiative on Psychiatry was founded in 1980 to combat the political abuse of psychiatry in the Soviet Union and other eastern European countries. It now works as a development agency working in mental health care in central and eastern Europe and the New Independent States (CCEE/NIS) and focuses its efforts on empowerment of local mental health reformers and their organizations (www. geneva-intitative.org).

2. In medicine a 'disease' has not only characteristic signs and symptoms (the 'syndrome') but also known underlying mechanisms and aetiologies. In psychiatry, most illness remains, in terms of classification, still at the level of the syndrome – with the exclusion of organic diseases with known aetiology, for example Alzeimer's disease – although considerable progress has been made in discovering abnormalities of brain functioning in other psychiatric illnesses.

3. There have been two large international comparative studies of people with a diagnosis of schizophrenia. In the WHO International Pilot Study of Schizophrenia (WHO 1973) it was established that the symptoms of people admitted to psychiatric hospitals in nine different countries were remarkably similar, despite major difference in language, religion, culture and degree of urbanization. A second study based on nearly 1,400 patients from twelve centres in ten countries demonstrated that the core symptoms of schizophrenia were again remarkably similar in all centres (Sartorius et al. 1986). See Littlewood (1996) and Kleinman (1991) for a critical discussion of these studies.

4. Roland Littlewood critically discusses these issues at much greater length in his paper (Littlewood 1996). Psychiatrists view the underlying biological processes (pathogenic factors) as determining the 'form' of symptoms which are common between cultures, and the personal and cultural factors (**pathoplastic** factors) as determining the 'content' of symptoms. For example *what* the person who is hearing voices hears the voices saying (content) is distinguished from the observation of the person that these voices speak *to each other* and *not directly to him* (form- *third* person auditory hallucinations which are a 'first rank' symptom of schizophrenia).

5. See Tyrer (1998: 360) who argues that community care is far from outmoded – 'Good community care is alive and well but it needs stimulation and succour.'

6. Christopher Clunis killed Jonathan Zito, a complete stranger, by stabbing him three times in the face while he waited for a train on the Piccadilly Line at Finsbury Park Station in the London Underground in 1992. The inquiry into the incident (Ritchie et al. 1994) found that Clunis suffered from paranoid schizophrenia and was undergoing community care and supervision from both psychiatric and social services at the time that he committed the offence, and revealed a 'catalogue of failure' in the care that Clunis had received.

5
THE FUTURE

Some cheerleaders and Cassandras

Cassandra was a prophetess in Greek mythology who foretold the outcome of many disastrous events in the ancient world. The earlier chapters of this book might lead the reader to the conclusion that the future of psychiatry is going to be overwhelmingly biological. Depending on your viewpoint, this might be an opportunity of great promise or a potential disaster for the profession. Whichever your perspective, the major concern of researchers within academic departments of psychiatry in North America and western Europe is now, undoubtedly, biologically oriented research. The subtitle of Nancy Andreasen's book, *Brave New Brain: Conquering Mental Illness in the Era of the Genome* (2001), seems to promise explicitly that embracing biology will provide us with that which doctors are always seeking – a cure. There is certainly no doubt that some developments will help doctors to tailor pharmacological treatment more precisely to the requirements of the individual patient. To cite one example (many would be possible, but reviewing advances in neurobiology is not the main purpose of this book), genetic variations in common liver enzymes have the potential to influence directly the efficacy and tolerability of commonly used psychotropic drugs. Studies are currently being carried out that will provide a step towards the individualization of drug treatment through enabling selection of the most beneficial drug according to the individual's genetic background (Arranz et al. 2001). The downside of this is, of course, that sensitive DNA information would be collected to predict response to medication – but might not always be used for this purpose. The implications of being known to be a 'non-responder' to specific drugs must also be considered.

David Healy, in his paper 'A dance to the music of the century', which appeared in the millennial edition of the *Psychiatric Bulletin*, used the opportunity to look back over the history of twentieth-century psychiatry, and specifically to criticize the way in which biology is being embraced:

> Where once blame had been put on families, or mothers in particular, the 1990s became the decade of blaming the brain (Valenstein 1998). By the end of the decade the psychobabble of yesteryear was fast being replaced by a newly minted biobabble. (Healy 2000: 2)

Healy's view of psychiatry in the new century is explicitly critical of the partnership between psychiatry and the pharmaceutical companies. But it does challenge us to question the prevalent biological agenda. In the same edition, Raj Persaud manages to embrace both the biological and the modernist vision, by contemplating a 'Big Brother' version of the future:

> Online monitoring of your physiology will enable managers in the future to know what kind of work you enjoy doing, and transmit more of this kind of work to your terminal. NHS administrators will better know which consultants are in fact sticking to their timetable by the activity coming from their desktops. Cure and relapse rates for each doctor, nurse and therapist's patient-load will be automatically fed back to staff and management so star practitioners can be easily identified, as well as those who will be automatically sent for more retraining and continued professional development. Hospital and physician league tables updated hourly will be available on the internet. (Persaud 2000a: 17)

While some of this monitoring of the practice of physicians and other therapists happens already, particularly in organizations such as **health maintenance organizations** in the USA, the practice of mental healthcare seems, by its very nature, to resist extreme attempts to control how it is carried out. In the USA (Goldman 2001) and in the UK (Kendell and Pearce 1997) psychiatrists have already voted with their feet by leaving systems of care that provide them with little opportunity to exercise either any degree of freedom in their clinical judgement or local interpretation of centralized planning initiatives.[1] In their contemplation of the state of American psychiatry, Hobson and Leonard quote a conversation with Daniel Weinburger, a distinguished psychiatrist and neurobiologist at the National Institute of Mental Health.

> Mental illness is a real thing. It's profoundly disabling and profoundly costly emotionally, psychologically, socially and economically to individuals and society. Psychiatry is the clinical discipline that has taken on the care of mental illness. Whether psychiatry disappears or is taken over by some subpopulation of neurologists or general medical doctors, there are going to be some people who have to care for the mentally ill, and there are certain unique skills that one has to learn....
>
> So there are going to have to be clinicians taking care of mentally ill people. Where do they do this? They can do it in HMOs, and they can be like any other doctor in that milieu. But if they are going to practice good

psychiatry and be effective in taking care of psychiatrically ill patients
they cannot be seeing a patient 15 minutes once every three months.
(Hobson and Leonard 2001: 210)

Such a scenario will be familiar to any psychiatrist working in the
UK National Health Service, and later in the chapter we will look
at ways clinicians are currently challenging this working pattern.

In a project that I carried out with Carl May and other colleagues
in Manchester (May et al. 2001), we explored the attitudes of mental health professionals to a telepsychiatry service and found a degree
of resistance to interviewing patients and service users across a vid-
eolink that one would not have predicted when browsing through
literature published by the enthusiasts of the new technology (for
example see Wootton et al. 2003). Raj Persaud's view of a medical
future apparently successfully driven by technology seems to me to
be as simplistic a vision of the future as one driven by genetics and
neuroimaging alone. Both leave the essential chaos of humanity
(professionals, patients and politicians) out of the equation.

A more balanced vision of the future was provided by the late
Robert Kendell (2000). Few would disagree with his view that over
the next twenty-five years we will see major advances in our understanding of the aetiology and pathogenesis of mental disorders. 'We
can be confident also that the major disorders that cause the most
disability are fundamentally disorders of cerebral function' (2000: 6).
But he tempers this statement thus: 'it is much harder though to
predict at what stage an increasing understanding of fundamental
mechanisms such as perception and memory will lead to major therapeutic advances' (ibid.: 7). He predicts that:

> Within the next decade or two a means will be found of preventing or
> delaying the deposition of amyloid.[2] When this happens the conse-
> quences for the image of old age psychiatry will be almost as profound as
> those for patients, their families and the nursing home industry. (ibid.: 7)

In Kendell's view psychiatry will become progressively more biological over the next twenty-five years, and less conceptually isolated
from medicine,

> as functional magnetic resonance imaging becomes a routine diagnostic
> tool, and changes in regional cerebral blood flow in response to mental
> tasks are measured in much the same way as electrocardiogram
> responses to exercise are monitored by cardiologists at present. (ibid.: 7)

But, as Kendell also points out, the rest of medicine may become
more aware of and interested in psychological and social influences
in morbidity and mortality. From my perspective as a teacher and

researcher in a medical school I see that, at the very time that psychiatry is becoming more biological and inevitably reductionist, developments in the rest of medicine, and particularly in medical education, are demanding that doctors be trained to be more 'holistic'. Traditionally it was to psychiatry that medical teachers turned for expertise in 'listening and talking to the patient', but no more. This place has undoubtedly been usurped by other medical educators, not least general practitioners. However, this causes concern among socially orientated psychiatrists, who see some of the stronger advocates of biology beginning to behave as though psychiatry will inevitably become little more than neuropsychiatry. I encountered this approach myself once at a hospital in North America when I asked the medical director his view of integration with psychiatry and he replied that it was all very straightforward. He wanted the psychiatry and neurology divisions to merge so that 'everything above the neck was together in the same place' (I think I have quoted him accurately). The attitudes of some neuropsychiatrists can also seem more reminiscent of the past than the future. As Tom Brown, who works as a liaison psychiatrist and therefore has generally progressive views about the integration of medicine and psychiatry, said to me: 'Biology has a lot to offer in the area of mental illness, but its links with the kind of alienism going back to a hundred years ago are still there.'

Yet the implicit influence of the biopsychosocial model can still be seen, for example, in recent research which aims to integrate aetiological models (for example Strickland et al. 2002).[3] Indeed many biological psychiatrists enthusiastically endorse the importance of psychosocial elements in both aetiology and treatment. As Bill Deakin said to me:

> I think what happens to you in early life is fantastically important. We are getting data about the effects of early physical and sexual abuse on your stress hormone responsiveness as an adult ... . In the neuroses there are information-processing biases that CBT can put right ... . I can see a time when it might be possible to do brain scans with psychological activation which will predict whether you're going to respond to drugs, or CBT or a combination of both.[4]

Now both psychiatrists and psychologists are seeking ways of linking together our new understanding of brain science with advances in clinical and experimental psychology (for examples see Hobson and Leonard (2001); or Bentall (2003) for a more sceptical perspective on the biological contribution to such a model). Leon Eisenberg, in a follow-up to his classic paper on 'mindlessness' and 'brainlessness' in psychiatry wisely comments that:

Biomedical knowledge is essential for providing sound medical care but it is not sufficient; the doctor's transactions with the patient must also be informed by psychosocial understanding. Neither mindlessness nor brainlessness can be tolerated in medicine. The unique role of psychiatry will be its contribution to a new paradigm, brain/mindfulness, integrating neurobiology with behaviour in its social context. That is the intellectual challenge ahead. (Eisenberg 2000: 4)

It seems to me that Eisenberg is asking psychiatry to move beyond the 'biopsychosocial model' to a new, more truly challenging integration of biological and cultural aspects of human behaviour, as envisaged by Kleinman (1991). According to Pilgrim (2002), in many teaching institutions the biopsychosocial model is now 'not so much opposed as treated with institutional cynicism' (2002: 73). Morris acknowledges the historical importance of the model but his approach revises the model in the light of post-modern thinking and proposes a new 'biocultural' perspective:

We must recognize that maladies, while always biological, are also in part cultural artefacts, in the same way that medicine is a cultural artefact as it operates through discourses that distribute social power across institutions and individual lives. (Morris 2000: 75)

According to Morris, psychiatric 'illnesses' such as depression are 'distinctive *postmodern* illnesses' in which there is a considerable interaction between biology and culture. However, within current psychiatric education there is still only limited reference to study of the culture of psychiatry itself, and of how the modern concepts of mental illness have been created during the last century (Horwitz 2002).

The revival of philosophical interest within psychiatry

This brings us to consider the upsurge, in recent years, of interest in philosophical and humanistic approaches to psychiatry, which is perhaps inevitable as a counterbalance to the increasing biological focus of psychiatric research. The arrival of 'post-psychiatry' with its focus on debate about contexts, values and partnerships, and argument that 'the voices of service users and survivors should now be centre stage' (Bracken and Thomas 2001: 727) can be seen as a marker of this shift. In the UK, the Royal College of Psychiatrists' Philosophy section is now the second largest in the college, with other similar groups appearing within professional associations across the world. In addition, the first Chair of Philosophy and Mental Health has been created at the University of Warwick. Bill

Fulford, who holds that chair, has proposed that this development
of a new philosophy of psychiatry, building on the work of Karl
Jaspers, is a 'permanent and positive shift in the intellectual climate
of psychiatry' (Fulford et al. 2003: 6). Fulford and his colleagues
argue that in articulating the things that make mental health more
difficult (rather than deficient) compared with other areas of health
care – the debates between different 'models' of mental illness and
between professional perspectives, the differences between cultural
presentations of mental illness, the often differing views of the
'users' of mental health services – we can lead the way for other
areas of health care.

In the same volume, Alfred Kraus (2003), Professor of Psychiatry
at Heidelberg, argues for a rediscovery of a 'phenomenological-
anthropological' (P-A) psychiatry, which he compares and contrasts
with the 'symptomatological-criteriological' (S-C) psychiatry inherent
in the modern classification system. He sees psychiatry as having
lost its way and discarded the original emphasis that Jaspers put on
the intuitive understanding of the other person's mental life by
empathic understanding. Through P-A approaches to diagnosis the
clinician puts particular weight on the patient's actual experiences:

> We try to understand the disturbance within the context of the whole
> person …. We try to understand a disturbance of thought or of mood in
> schizophrenia and mania by an alteration of the whole 'being in the
> world' of the person concerned. (Kraus 2003: 205)

This approach demands a very different sort of relationship between
the patient and the clinician, in which the patient is not merely a
'supplier of data' but a collaborator, and not 'merely a bearer of
symptoms, as the object or victim of an illness' (Kraus 2003: 213).
This approach seeks to reinforce the original message of Jaspers –
that meanings as well as causes are essential to good clinical care.[5]

If it is to survive and make a lasting impact on psychiatry, it is
essential that this new philosophy of psychiatry tackles the conceptual difficulties inherent in the practical everyday work of the profession. We have already explored some of these practical difficulties
in earlier chapters, in particular the threats posed by legislation
which appears to be seeking to use psychiatry for the purposes of
social control. However, the brave new world (not surprising, perhaps, with the echoes of Aldous Huxley) visualized by Andreasen in
Brave New Brain brings with it numerous ethical dilemmas for the
practising clinician. There are many ways in which the principles of
respect for individual persons may be eroded in the face of a new
'scientific' certainty. Andreasen (2001: 338) ponders the implications

of research briefly ('will the growth of biomedical technology dehumanize psychiatry?') but ultimately concludes with a positivist message about 'unparalleled opportunities to reduce suffering'. To me, this seems both unduly simplistic and a failure to recognize and grasp the challenge. At the coal face, practising clinicians will find themselves facing an increasing range of ethical challenges, from informing people about the results of screening for carrier status of genetic risk for mental illness (something faced already with Huntington's disease), to the role that the psychiatrist may be asked to take in decision-making about sanctioning assisted suicide for a person with terminal illness (Kelly and McLoughlin 2002) – currently a topical issue in western countries. The psychiatrist of the future will not be able to rely on tacit acceptance of his or her decisions made for others, regardless of whether or not they were made 'in good faith'.

Specialists and generalists

Over the last quarter-century, the practice of medicine has become more specialized. It is unusual now, outside of primary care, to find a physician who considers him or herself to be a generalist. Physicians are increasingly specializing in different branches of medicine and those fields are becoming narrower. This trend began in the USA, which has always allowed direct access of patients to specialist care, but has also extended to countries where the general practitioner acts as gatekeeper to the specialist, such as the UK. It is also now extending to physicians who become psychiatrists. Part of the problem increasingly facing psychiatrists, as with other medical practitioners, is the sheer amount of knowledge and variety of differing skills, across a number of different fields, they need to acquire during training. Weissman et al. (1999) have put forward the view that one reason for the apparent inability of practitioners to embrace the biopsychosocial model in everyday clinical work is that psychiatrists are not adequately trained to master all the sub-disciplines required. We have seen, in an earlier chapter, how training in psychotherapy is undergoing revision in the UK. As yet, psychiatrists have not routinely been educated in many of the other cultural and philosophical concepts that I have discussed in this chapter and this poses a considerable educational challenge to those of us in the profession who regularly teach. Nevertheless, it seems to have been easier for psychiatrists, for many of the reasons discussed in earlier chapters of this book, to become specialists in biological aspects of mental health care rather than in social and psychological aspects. As Robert Kendell noted (2000), even though eminent psychiatrists (such as Aaron Beck and Isaac Marks) were central to the development of the new psychotherapies, these highly effective therapies have now, largely, been taken over by clinical psychologists and (to an increasing degree) by nurses. As a result it is now these professions that are seen as the main exponents of evidence-based and cost-effective psychotherapies.

A current issue facing psychiatrists in the UK, as we saw in Chapter 3, is dissatisfaction with the working pattern and clinical role of the 'general psychiatrist' who sees a wide range of front-line clinical problems. Typically, the general psychiatrist has responsibility for a sector or 'patch', which might be a defined geographical area or a group of patients registered with a specific list of general practitioners who work in a particular part of a town or city. The general psychiatrist's role is increasingly stressful. There is a strongly felt perception that the division of work between general psychiatry and its sub-specialities has been unfairly developed and maintained (Kennedy and Griffiths 2001), with rehabilitation, forensic psychiatry, substance misuse and psychological therapy services being set up with unilaterally defined limits. The patients these specialists do not wish to see are considered the responsibility of the generalist. Forensic psychiatrists see offering psychiatric assessment and treatment to people with mental health problems passing through the courts (court-diversion schemes) as the role of general psychiatrists. The same is increasingly the case with the psychiatric care of people already within the prison service – which has hitherto always been the remit of forensic services. Jenny Shaw, Senior Lecturer in Forensic Psychiatry told me: 'General psychiatry has tried to shunt some of the more difficult clients upwards into forensic services and gradually over time forensic services have expanded more and more, taking areas that perhaps should be done by general psychiatrists.' Jenny says the role of forensic psychiatry is much narrower: 'It's the very heavy end of the market, the very serious offences' (interviewed 2003).

The attraction of training for a specific speciality in psychiatry is that it brings a more defined role, often (as with forensic and elderly services) increasing investment from the government, and a much less 'front-line' role than general psychiatry. Dinesh Bhugra comments:

Maybe the time has come to abolish general psychiatry as a specialism and go by what the physicians have done, by illnesses, ... so that GPs become general psychiatrists and make the diagnosis and send them to the schizophrenia specialist or whatever. Professor X [a famous London psychiatrist] has always been very fond of saying that sooner or later psychosis is going to be hived off to CPNs, neurosis would go to CBT and psychology, and personality disorder would go to forensic, and general psychiatry would be left with what nobody else wants! (Interviewed 2003)

However, I agree with the view that specialists can only exist, by definition, when there is a healthy generalist service acting as gate-keeper (Mathers and Hodgkin 1989; Deahl and Turner 1997) and, to those us of who work closely with general practitioners, it seems there is neither widespread enthusiasm, the necessary front-line support, nor the expertise ever to take on the generalist function from the general psychiatrist in British psychiatry. Maybe patients always want to see the 'expert', but Mike Shooter, the UK College President, thinks that patients also want to know there is someone who knows the whole story, and it isn't good enough to say: 'Oh it will be the GP.' People who use psychiatric services have told him that they 'want to be held by somebody along that path, somebody needs to stay close to me'. In an era of ever more fragmented and specialized care this is harder to achieve.

Various ideas are currently being discussed for improving the lot of the generalist in psychiatry. Dinesh Bhugra, who has been very active in the Royal College of Psychiatrists in the section of General Adult Psychiatry, discussed with me the possibilities that have been mooted for generalists – particularly those who work in the stressful and very demanding inner-city setting – having smaller populations for which to provide care, sharing responsibilities with one or more consultants for a sector instead of working alone, and working for a limited period at the front line, perhaps for a period of five years, before moving on to another job. Peter Kennedy and Hugh Griffiths (2001) have considered new approaches to the job description of the generalist which involve much more delegation to other mental health workers, and an end to 'routine' outpatient clinics, so that the consultant can respond in support of other professionals in deal-ing with crises. However, discussion of new roles has been accom-panied by concerns about what this reconsideration of the 'consultant' role actually means in practice. The shortage of psychi-atrists tends to reinforce the traditional role of supervision carried out by the consultant in the medical profession as the 'senior specialist'. According to Timms (2003), however, it implies not only 'a portfolio of privileges we no longer enjoy', but is also in conflict with our everyday practice, which seems to be what our customers (and the government) want – that is, direct provision of care, face to face with the patient in a 'consultant-delivered service' (Department of Health 2000). Mike Shooter expressed it thus:

Looking at creative ways of working for consultants, the biggest anxiety most keenly expressed has been 'will this be just another way of promoting me away from what I want to do and what I do best, which is actually working with individual patients, groups of patients their families and their carers?' (Interviewed 2003)

But he is optimistic about the future: 'If I was starting again as a trainee I'd want to be a general adult psychiatrist because I think that's where the creativity is going to occur in the next five to ten years.' Understanding the potential for this creative explosion lies in considering how the psychiatrist of the future can find his or her unique role in the community, not just of mental health professionals, but also in relation to the patient or user of mental health services.

The role of the psychiatrist in mental health care

Psychiatry is a medical discipline that is concerned with the recognition and treatment of mental disorders. It is important to recall that there is a distinction between psychiatry and mental health programmes. Mental health programmes are broader than psychiatry and somewhat different in their nature. (Sartorius 2002: 94)[6]

Many professionals other than psychiatrists are involved in the design, planning and delivery of a comprehensive system of mental health care. Other mental health professionals, including psychiatrists, working partly or entirely in the private sector, play a role in the complex jigsaw of mental health care provision. Sartorius goes on to say that 'it is obvious that many psychiatrists will concentrate on the recognition and treatment of mental disorders. They will want to have an independent discipline unencumbered by the need to deal with diseases other than those that have been labelled psychiatric'(2002: 3). However, he goes on to point out that: 'Some [of the world's 150,000 psychiatrists] are constantly, and almost painfully aware of the fact that they can only deal with a minute proportion of people with mental illnesses' (ibid.: 4). The majority of people with mental health problems worldwide are not helped by mental health specialists of any variety, but by general health workers and a variety of lay supporters.

In public health systems in some countries of the developing world, notably the UK and Australia, the focus of psychiatry has narrowed even further, to people defined as having 'severe and enduring mental illness' (which is most commonly interpreted by the health care system as meaning primarily schizophrenia, organic brain disease and bipolar disorder).[7] From the viewpoint of the profession this has advantages. One such advantage is a defined focus for work, which fits both with the economic drive to contain the costs of specialist health care and with the interest of biological orientation in that these are 'diseases' that can be reliably diagnosed and investigated using the new research methodologies of neuroimaging. But, for some, this represents a retreat into the past, which relates to the new emphasis on building secure facilities to protect the public. Tom Brown's views echo my own:

> Psychiatry is retreating into alienism and going back to the asylum days where all we see are mad people. I am appalled at the use of the term 'severe and enduring mental illness' – to some extent I think politicians and a lot of psychiatrists have colluded in a narrow interpretation, politicians for reasons of money and safety and psychiatrists to contain their workload. A few years down the line we have a generation of psychiatrists who, faced with a patient who is not psychotic, haven't got a clue what to do. It's damaging to the speciality that people even contest the status of recurrent major depression as a severe and enduring mental illness. (Interviewed 2003)

In terms of the total burden of mental ill-health in the world two sources of data should be borne in mind. First, the much-quoted World Bank report that depression is estimated to be the fourth largest contributor to the global burden of disease (Murray and Lopez, 1995), and by 2020 is projected to become the single largest in developing regions. Second, the view that half the disability associated with mental disorders worldwide is generated by anxiety and the affective disorders, and less than 10 per cent by schizophrenia (Andrews 2000). Gavin Andrews comments that the spending on mental health care is actually the converse of this in his native Australia (as in the UK), with the bulk of expenditure going on the care of psychotic illness. Nevertheless, from an economic perspective, 'the bottom line is really the efficiency of the interventions in reducing mortality and morbidity' (ibid.: 20), and research cannot yet provide us with the answer to this question. Perhaps it is cynical to point out that a considerable amount of the cost of managing people with a diagnosis of schizophrenia both in Australia and in the UK goes on meeting the salaries of the psychiatrists. But Carl May, Professor of Medical Sociology in Newcastle, sees problems for the future of the profession if it pursues a narrow, biological role in the management of psychosis:

> If it genuinely is about which receptor system needs to be adjusted, what bit of brain needs to be tweaked by the pharmaceutical companies then I can't see why it requires somebody paid whatever a consultant psychiatrist is paid to make that decision .... There could easily be a new kind of physician's assistant who trains in interpreting material. (Interviewed 2003)

When routine technical work is increasingly devolved to nurses who, it is well known, are better than doctors at implementing protocol-driven care, psychiatrists may begin to seem an expensive option in publicly funded systems. This is quite apart from the impact Carl May believes this focus of work might ultimately have on recruitment: 'If in the end a group of clinicians only attract the most difficult and intractable patients and rarely see patients whom they can do anything positive for, then this seems to me to be a very depressing scenario.' Mental health professionals who devote their life to working with people with 'treatment-resistant' illness may be appalled by this statement, but it does echo the concerns expressed earlier in Chapter 3 about recruitment of medical students into psychiatry, and the problems faced by those general psychiatrists who are gradually building up large case-loads of people 'with whom individual members of the Community Mental Health Team say they cannot cope' (Kennedy and Griffiths 2001: 283).

Other psychiatrists, coming from the public health perspective of Sartorius and taking a 'population-based' approach (see Box 6) to the management of mental health problems in the community, have a much broader view of the psychiatrist of the future. Greg Simon is a distinguished psychiatric researcher, who has carried out research over many years at the Center for Health Studies in Seattle, into improving the quality of care for people with mental health problems in primary care. He sees the need for a shift in the role of psychiatrists to one of working collaboratively with other mental health professionals and primary care physicians, to improve the quality of care for people in a defined population who suffer from mental illness. Specific 'stepped-care' (see Box 7) pathways from primary into specialist care would be supported not only with protocols to govern the content of treatment, but also effective case management, timely support from specialists for supervision and consultation, and transfer to exclusive specialist treatment only for people with more complex or treatment-resistant illness.

The psychiatrist will act as an educator of others as well as supervisor, collaborator (with other professionals) and advocate (for meeting the needs of those with mental health problems).[8] This seems to provide a possible future model not only for the 'generalist specialist' within psychiatry, as the professional who links most closely with primary care, but also for those psychiatrists who work within particular specialities as different as drug dependence and assertive outreach, where liaison with professionals working on other 'steps' in care provision is necessary in order to provide the right type of care to the right person at the right time. The psychiatrist,

---

Box 6   A population-based approach to care

Development and implementation of a structured strategy for care for all patients in a defined population with a recurrent or chronic illness.

Population based care is not simply 'public health' – but is clinically focused on *improvement of quality of care.*

Box 7   The concept of 'stepped care'

Stepped care as applied to 'depression':

- Targets patients who fail to recover after initial management by the primary care physician and patients who are at high risk of relapse.

- Targets more intensive interventions (e.g. cognitive behaviour therapy, expert pharmacotherapy by psychiatrist) to patients who do not achieve a favourable outcome after an initial less intensive intervention.

---

with his or her broad range of expertise across the biocultural spectrum, has a key part to play, as summarized by Mike Shooter:

> I think it's something to do with the ability to understand a lot of possible components of a person's problem, of a family's situational problem and be able to take stock of all of those components simultaneously, to contain the anxiety of the situation and yet be able to act in an emergency when necessary and to hold that anxiety while you're taking stock and working out which of those components is the most important to address and what's needed. And I think there really is something about the diagnostic process, in the true sense of the word, which is a unique part of medical training. I don't think we should be humble about that.

The phrase 'working in partnership' has become something of a cliché in the last few years, but survival of a healthy and successful psychiatric profession must depend on its ability to work in an environment of genuine collaboration, both with other mental health professionals and with the people themselves who use the mental health services. From a public health perspective there is plenty of work to do, and we have to be able to get along with each other to achieve it. This takes time, effort and space for conversation to change attitudes and preconceptions (for example those of psychiatrists about psychologists and vice versa), and also to address those fears and anxieties that patients have about psychiatrists, notwithstanding the somewhat negative views that some psychiatrists still hold about the 'user movement'. I wholeheartedly disagree with Dorothy Rowe (see page 91) when she criticizes those psychiatrists who work hard to integrate not just within the profession but across its boundaries, but I will continue both to acknowledge and to try and understand her point of view! And I will conclude with a final word from Mike Shooter:

> I want to be remembered as the person who took us into the Mental Health Alliance, on one side the users' and carers' organizations and, on the other, the other organizations in the mental health world, because I think we stand or fall together. (Mike Shooter, President of the Royal College of Psychiatrists interviewed by the author 2003)

Notes

1. Mental health policy in England and Wales was overhauled at the end of the 1990s by the publication of the National Service Framework for mental health (NHSE 1999) and the NHS National Plan (Department of Health 2000), which sets clear centrally determined targets for the number and type of services that must be provided by mental health trusts. Similar policy documents were published for Scotland. Further upheaval is under way with the consultation over the revised Mental Health Act (Scotland already has a new Mental Health Act).

2. Microscopic plaques of amyloid (a protein) are a characteristic pathological feature in the brains of people with a diagnosis of Alzheimer's disease.

3. Paul Strickland and colleagues (Strickland et al. 2002) attempted to explore whether social adversity might be a risk factor for depression by increasing cortisol secretion, which impairs serotonin (5HT) neurotransmission. They examined this possible causal pathway – linking biological and social factors in the aetiology of depression, in a community sample in South Manchester. However, they concluded that although the **HPA axis** is sensitive to social stress it did not mediate vulnerability to depression.

4. He did temper this with the rider: 'It's typical hand-waving biological psychiatry promissory stuff!'

5. For a critical review of the place of Jaspers in the history of 'defining madness' see Bentall (2003). Bentall suggests that by introducing the empathetic but extremely subjective test of 'understandability' into the diagnostic process (if content of the patient's ideas is 'ununderstandable' the patient must be psychotic), Jaspers actually discouraged further psychological research into psychosis and 'inadvertently gave madness to the biologists' (2003: 29). It seems to me that the advances in biological psychiatry about the structural and neurological abnormalities to be found in the brains of people with a diagnosis of schizophrenia have been far more important in the apparent 'takeover' by the biological psychiatrists. Indeed, in mid-twentieth-century American psychiatry (where the biological swing has been the greatest) psycho-analysis was widely employed as a treatment for psychosis. I would agree with Bentall that effective psychological treatments are now available, but unfortunately they are not *widely* available.

6. According to Sartorius, mental health programmes are:

> Aggregates of activities designed to (i) promote mental health, (ii) prevent mental illness, (iii) ensure the treatment of the mentally ill, (iv) rehabilitate

those who are disabled by mental disorders and (v) provide technical support to efforts aiming to diminish psychosocial problems such as the erosion of families in conditions of rapid social change. (Sartorius 2002: 94–95)

7. Despite general agreement that 'severe and enduring mental illness' should be defined in terms of disability and severity of symptoms, many professionals within UK health and social care still apply, on a day-to-day basis, a diagnostic test when overseeing access to services such as specialist mental health care.

8. I mean here to distinguish this type of advocacy, which is really a kind of political sensibility and willingness to engage in debate about policy, from the advocacy services provided for users of mental health services (see Thomas and Bracken 1999) which seek to represent the views of users of psychiatric services and, by their very nature, should stand apart from the professions. In advocating for the rights of people with mental health problems it is, however, essential that one does not fall into the trap of paternalistically 'knowing what is needed'. This is one of the reasons why attempting to work with the organizations that seek to represent the views of patients is so important. But it is also important to try to understand empathically not just the symptoms but also the experience of receiving health care in the organization in which you work, from the perspective of a patient being treated there, as well as from your own as an employee.

Appendices

APPENDIX 1

INFORMATION ON PSYCHIATRY AS A CAREER (REPRINTED WITH PERMISSION FROM THE ROYAL COLLEGE OF PSYCHIATRISTS WEBSITE: WWW.RCPSYCH.AC.UK)

You must first qualify as a medical doctor. To do this, you need to be accepted by a medical school, having passed three good 'A' levels in subjects such as Chemistry, Zoology, Physics, Biology or Maths. Some medical schools now accept other 'A' levels, too. Getting into medical school is very competitive – it seems to help if candidates not only have good academic qualifications but are also lively, enthusiastic all-rounders with outside interests such as sports or the Arts.

Once you have been accepted by a hospital as a medical student, you will work in a variety of areas, including psychiatry, for the next five years.

Following this, you will work as a House Officer in a hospital for a further year. This can be very tough with hard work and long hours. However, once you get through this, you will become a medical doctor and can specialize in any area you wish – we hope you will choose psychiatry!

Before starting your psychiatric training, we advise young doctors to take an extra job or two in the general medicine or Accident and Emergency departments of a hospital – this always seems to help during your first psychiatric job.

You will then spend a further three years working as a Senior House Officer – during which time you will probably wish to study for the Royal College of Psychiatrists' Membership Examination – the MRCPsych.

Following this, you will be ready for Higher Training as a Specialist Registrar. During this period, you will choose which of the six psychiatric speciality areas you wish to concentrate upon during the next three/four years.

What are the various specialties within psychiatry?

General adult psychiatry
The majority of psychiatrists in the UK work within this broad category, which involves the care of people with mental health problems

in many settings. Psychiatrists may be based in mental or university hospitals, psychiatric units in general hospitals, in the community, or a mixture of these. Because of the diversity of patients and psychiatric conditions requiring treatment and care, an adult general psychiatrist must be skilled in numerous treatment techniques. Psychiatrists in this area must also have the knowledge and skills required to organize and administer a psychiatric service for a specific population. General adult psychiatrists may have a special interest in, for example, neuropsychiatry, the rehabilitation and care of patients with chronic disabilities, drug and/or alcohol problems or eating disorders. They work closely with multi-disciplinary teams which can include community psychiatric nurses, social workers, psychologists and occupational therapists. This specialty also entails close liaison with hostels, crisis intervention centres, residential homes and sheltered workshops.

Psychiatry of old age

This is a rapidly expanding specialty: the number of old people in this country has increased dramatically, and is likely to continue to do so. In psychiatric units at present, about 45 per cent of residents and 25 per cent of people admitted are aged 65 years or more. A major challenge for this area of psychiatry is the treatment and care of people suffering from senile dementia, but most specialists in the field deal with the full range of psychiatric disorders affecting patients over the age of 65. Much ill health in old people is a mixture of physical and mental conditions, and so an active interest in general medicine is required. Psychiatrists working in this specialty are based in hospitals, geriatric units, day-care centres, or in the community. Experience in general medicine, geriatrics, general practice and psychology is particularly valuable.

Child and adolescent psychiatry

Psychiatrists working in this area are primarily concerned with the intellectual, emotional and behavioural mental health problems of children from birth until school-leaving age. The development of a close working relationship with the child concerned – and their family – is essential. Skills in diagnostic assessment, including interviewing and examination, are particularly valuable. You would use a variety of treatments ranging from individual psychotherapy to behavioural and family therapy. You could be based in hospitals, child guidance clinics, day units, special schools (boarding and day) for children experiencing difficulties, or in community and remand homes. It may also be necessary to engage in Court activities.

Forensic psychiatry
This is concerned with the interaction between and overlap with psychiatry and the law. The forensic psychiatrist cares for and treats offenders with mental health problems in a number of different settings: general and special hospitals, crisis intervention centres, and prisons.

In addition, forensic psychiatrists work with the courts in the elucidation of medico-legal problems such as criminal responsibility, fitness to plead and the management of mentally abnormal offenders.

Special skills are needed in assessing behavioural abnormalities, understanding and using security as a means of control and treatment, writing reports for Courts and lawyers and giving evidence in Courts of law.

Forensic psychiatry is challenging, since it sometimes involves dealing with very disturbed patients, who may have violent tendencies.

Psychiatry of learning disability (formerly mental handicap)
Psychiatrists working in this area are concerned with the prevention, diagnosis and treatment of the mental health problems which often occur in people with learning disability. For example, a patient with Down's Syndrome may also suffer from depression or anxiety. Psychiatrists in this area work closely with the patient's family, taking into consideration their care and education. In addition to psychiatric and administrative skills, expertise in related subjects such as paediatrics, neurology, genetics, biochemistry and psychology are required. To an increasing extent, learning disability psychiatrists work in teams based in special schools and training centres, hospitals, residential hostels and sheltered workshops.

Psychotherapy
All psychiatrists need some basic psychotherapeutic skills, but specialists in this area are also required to assess and treat people with, for example, psychoneuroses, personality and behavioural disorders, and sexual and interpersonal problems. In addition to specialized treatment procedures, psychotherapists need expertise in the application of psychotherapeutic principles, including the psychodynamic use of the doctor–patient relationship as part of the general management of all patients with mental health and psychosomatic disorders.

Psychotherapists also need to be skilled in cognitive and behavioural therapies. During training, it may be necessary to experience personal psychotherapy. This gives psychiatrists a valuable insight into their patients' problems.

An increasing number of psychotherapists work closely with various clinical teams in hospitals, child and adolescent units, child guidance clinics, student health centres, and in doctors' surgeries.

Are there opportunities for psychiatrists wishing to work in the Armed Forces?

Yes. Psychiatrists in the Armed Forces provide help with mental health problems to about 500,000 men, women and children in the UK and overseas. In addition to Service personnel, those entitled to benefit from the Defence Medical Services include civilians employed by the Ministry of Defence overseas (such as schoolteachers, welfare professionals, shopkeepers and administrative staff) and the families of Service personnel and other entitled civilians.

Military psychiatrists are trained as general adult psychiatrists. They may have a special interest in the maintenance of fitness and morale, and in the study of combat stress, both physical and psychological. Service psychiatrists are based more and more in the community, and are supported by community psychiatric nurses or social workers.

All doctors working within the Armed Forces enlist as military personnel, and undergo some general military training. Before starting specialist psychiatric training, it is usual for Service doctors to spend one or two years undertaking general medical duties to enable them to acquire an understanding of the conditions of life among the Armed Forces.

How is training organized?

General training

During your general training in a medical school – lasting approximately 5–6 years – you could choose an 'elective' period in psychiatry (about 3–4 months). You would then carry on working in pre-registration posts (i.e. House Officer posts) for a period of one year. After this, you become registered with the General Medical Council (GMC). In your post-registration period working as a Senior House Officer, you should try to gain experience recognized by the Royal College of Psychiatrists, such as working in general practice or general medicine.

Basic specialist training

Your basic specialist training in psychiatry takes place on College-approved and recognized Rotational Training Schemes, and lasts three years; you would spend about six months each in as many specialties as are offered by the training scheme – as well as fulfilling the basic requirement to train (initially for one year) in general adult and old age psychiatry. You should ensure that your particular area of interest, i.e. psychotherapy or forensic, is covered by your training scheme. Details of recognized training schemes are available from the College on request. After initial training, and at least one year's experience of general psychiatry, you would be ready to sit for Part I of the College Membership examination – the MRCPsych.

The MRCPsych (Membership) examination

The emphasis of the Membership exam is on clinical work:

Part I consists of a Multiple Choice Question (MCQ) Paper and a clinical examination which will be a test of clinical skills in assessment.

Part I must be passed within three years of full-time approved psychiatric training (or equivalent period of part-time training).

Part II consists of a second clinical examination, much broader than the first, two MCQ papers, an Essay Paper and a paper containing questions on basic sciences and clinical topics.

Once you have successfully obtained Part I, you should work as an SHO in rotating specialty posts for a further 2/3 years, after which time you would be eligible to take Part II of the examination. If you pass, you are awarded the MRCPsych, and become a Member of the College. To summarize, to obtain the MRCPsych, you would need:

- a minimum of one year's psychiatric experience before taking the Part I
- two to three years' further training before taking the Part II (although this period can be shorter if you have other training that is recognized by the College, such as general practice medicine, general medicine, etc). Full details are available on request from the Examinations Department of the College.

Higher specialist training

Higher specialist training entails working as a Specialist Registrar or Lecturer for a further three/four years. During higher specialist training, there is an opportunity to work in general adult psychiatry, or you can opt for one of the specialties as listed above, with a special interest in another sub-specialty such as forensic or liaison psychiatry. After completion of higher specialist training, you could apply for posts such as Senior Lecturer, Consultant or Professor of Psychiatry.

Further information is available from:
Gareth Holsgove
Head of Postgraduate Educational Services
The Royal College of Psychiatrists
17 Belgrave Square
London SW1X 8PG (email: gholsgrove@rcpsych.ac.uk)

Flow chart of training as a psychiatrist in the UK and Eire

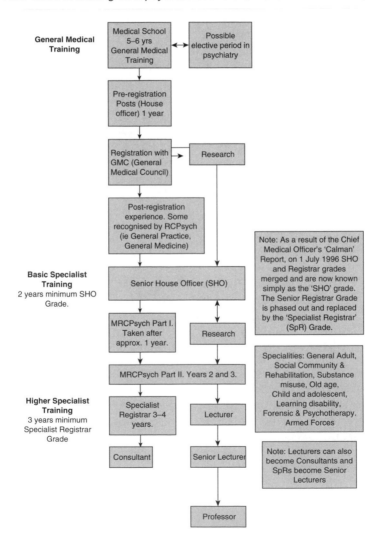

APPENDIX 2
GLOSSARY OF SOME TERMS USED IN THE TEXT

Affective disorders: disorders characterized by a primary disturbance of mood such as depression or elation. Depression often co-exists with anxiety in the community although anxiety disorders are classified separately.

Amnesia: loss of memory.

Anorexia: loss of appetite. This occurs in many physical and mental disorders (e.g. depression) and should be distinguished from the eating disorder *anorexia nervosa* in which there is deliberate restriction of food intake, weight loss, disturbed body image and amenorrhoea. Anorexia nervosa is traditionally viewed as a 'neurotic' illness even though the behaviour of a person with the disorder may seem to defy the test of 'understandability' and therefore seem to have more in common with psychotic thinking (see Jaspers 1913).

Assertive Community Treatment: provision of community-based, multidisciplinary care to individuals with long-standing psychiatric illnesses who have previously been, or are at risk of, hospitalization. ACT services are flexible and support people who may have a history of non-engagement with treatment.

Aversion therapy: negative conditioning. The unwanted behaviour (for example alcohol abuse, sexual deviation) is paired with painful or unpleasant stimuli until it is extinguished.

Barbiturates: a group of drugs that are central nervous system depressants. Widely prescribed in the past for insomnia, they are now rarely prescribed for this reason, because of serious problems with addiction and lethality in overdose.

Bipolar disorder: affective disorder characterized by episodes of both mania and depression. Also known as manic-depressive psychosis but this term is now much less used.

Catatonic schizophrenia: one of the sub-groups of schizophrenia characterized by the presence of one or more states of abnormal movement such as stupor (unresponsiveness with immobility and mutism but retention of consciousness), maintenance of rigid postures or facial expressions (grimacing) or idiosyncratic involuntary movements (known as mannerisms). For a fuller description see Sims (2003).

Cognitive-behaviour therapy (CBT): an active, structured, directive and time-limited therapy which is based on the belief that the way a person perceives himself, the world and the future determines his mood and his behaviour. The therapy has both cognitive (focusing on identification and challenging of negative thoughts) and behavioural (focusing on goal-setting and behavioural activation) components.

Comorbid (comorbidity): occurrence of more than one disease in the same time in the same person. More popular as a concept in American than in European traditions of psychiatric diagnosis and classification.

Culture-bound syndromes: syndromes (characteristic patterns of symptoms and behaviour) that appear to be limited to certain societies or cultures.

Degeneration: the notion that inherited mental illness worsened steadily over the generations – causing progressive deterioration within families and within the population as a whole. This idea was popular within nineteenth-century psychiatry. It is but one step, however, from applying eugenic principles to improve the genetic stock – the path pursued by the Nazis.

Delusion: a false, unshakeable idea or belief which is out of keeping with the person's educational, cultural and social background.

Dementia praecox: term coined by Morel in 1857 to describe psychoses with a poor prognosis (deterioration or 'dementia') which often begin in early life (praecox). Kraepelin differentiated psychosis with a better prognosis (manic-depressive psychosis) from dementia praecox which later became generally known as schizophrenia (see below).

Desensitization: a form of behaviour therapy which is particularly effective in treatment of phobia.

Electro-convulsive therapy (ECT): the treatment of mental disorders, most commonly severe depression, by passing an electric current through the brain with the use of general anaesthesia and a muscle relaxant.

Electronarcosis: obsolete early variety of ECT.

Flooding: effective behavioural treatment for phobia which involves prolonged exposure to the situation which is avoided.

General systems theory: a movement in scientific theory which sought to discover general patterns, trends and structural characteristics in all types of system – natural, social and technological. It was a reaction against the fragmented acquisition of knowledge resulting from excessive specialization.

Hallucination: an apparent perception of an external object when no such object is present. Hallucinations may be experienced in all the sensory domains – visual, auditory, tactile and olfactory.

Health Maintenance Organizations (HMOs): organized health care delivery system to be found in the USA which provides enrollees with comprehensive health care (which may be limited for certain illnesses – particularly mental illnesses) for a fixed term in return for regular payment of premiums.

Huntington's disease: inherited neuropsychiatric disorder which results in progressive disability from disorders of movement (chorea), depression and dementia.

Hypothalamo–pituitary–adrenal (HPA) axis: part of the endocrine system (hormones) which plays an important part in coping with stress. The hypothalamus and pituitary gland are located in the brain and the adrenal glands just above the kidneys. When a person is under stress the hypothalamus triggers the pituitary to release a hormone which finally triggers the adrenals to release cortisol. Many people with mood disorders appear to have a cortisol regulation system which is not working effectively.

Hysteria: old-fashioned term for dissociative (conversion) disorder which implies the behaviour of illness (for example paralysis of a limb) without evidence of physical pathology. There is continued debate about the usefulness of the term – see Sims (2003) for a comprehensive discussion.

Insulin coma treatment: obsolete treatment which involved the induction of coma through the administration of insulin.

Leucotomy, lobotomy: psychosurgical procedure which involved destruction of an area of brain tissue. Still performed for intractable illnesses in a small number of specialist centres.

Loosening of associations: a type of disorder of the expression of thought in speech, in which there is incompleteness of the development of ideas. The person's conversation sounds muddled and their thoughts seem to veer off until they may appear unrelated to whatever apparently initiated them.

Managed behavioural healthcare organization (MBHO): an organized system of behavioural health care delivery – usually to a defined population of members of **HMOs** and other **managed care** structures. Also known as a 'carve-out'. See Talbott and Hales (2001) for more detailed description.

Managed care: the general term used to describe a variety of arrangements in health care financing, organization and delivery in which an entity other than the directly treating physician is managing or over-seeing payments for medical services. The commonest type of managed care programme separates mental health provision from general health provision, with mental health care being provided by a large behavioural health organization. This split of the physical from the mental once again perpetuates Cartesian dualism through the justification of twentieth-century economics.

Manic-depressive psychosis: see **bipolar disorder**.

Mental state examination: the psychiatric equivalent of the physical examination which seeks to create a record of behavioural and psychological data elicited by examination at the time of the interview as well as by contemporaneous observation. Data are traditionally recorded under the headings: appearance and general behaviour, talk or speech, mood, thought content (including abnormal beliefs and perceptions), cognitive state and insight (see Goldberg and Murray, *The Maudsley Handbook of Practical Psychiatry* (2002), which is a widely used text for psychiatric trainees).

Mono-Amine Oxidase Inhibitors (or **MAOIs**): early type of antidepressant. Rarely used now because of potentially dangerous interactions with certain foods and numerous other drugs.

Neuroimaging: brain imaging is a computer-assisted graphic representation of brain structure. Methods used include X-ray computerized axial tomography (CT or CAT scanning), NMR (nuclear magnetic resonance, which uses magnetic field instead of radiation to produce images), PET (positron emission tomography, which employs chemicals tagged with radio-isotopes) and SPECT (single photon emission computed tomography, which uses radiopharmaceutical agents or radioactive gas).

Neuroleptic: a drug which has a specific anti-psychotic effect and is not simply achieving its effect by tranquillization.

Neuroradiological/neuroradiologists: the study of the brain originally using X-rays but now involving a wide variety of imaging techniques (see **neuroimaging**).

Obsessional neurosis/obsessive-compulsive disorder: a disorder characterized by persistent, disturbing, unwanted, anxiety-provoking, intruding thoughts, ideas, images and/or impulses to perform repetitive acts (rituals). Typically the person regards these as alien or absurd.

Pathoplastic: pathoplastic factors change the way in which an illness presents; for example, cultural factors commonly do this even if they do not actually cause the illness in the first place.

Phenomenology: the study of events in their own right, rather than from the point of view of inferred causes. In psychiatry it is specifically:

> The observation and categorization of abnormal psychological events, the internal experiences of the patient and his consequent behaviour. An attempt is made to observe and understand the psychological event or phenomenon, so that the observer can, as far as possible, know for himself what the patient's experience must feel like. (Sims 2003: 3)

Phobias: unreasonable and inappropriate fears.

Psychiatric genetics: study of the inheritance of biological variation as it pertains to the aetiology of psychiatric illnesses.

Psychodynamic (or psychoanalytically orientated) psychotherapy: psychotherapy theoretically rooted in the ideas of Freud and those who followed him. Based on theories which represent symptomatic behaviour as determined by the interplay between intra- and extra-psychic forces (for example family conflict, early experiences, current life stresses).

Psychoneuroendocrinologists/psychoneuroendocrinology: study of the endocrine system as a likely site for biochemical abnormalities that are significant in the aetiology of psychiatric illnesses. Recent research has focused on the central regulatory actions of the **HPA axis**.

Psychopharmacology: the study of the behavioural effects of drugs.

Psychosurgery: the use of (neuro)surgical means to treat mental illness.

Randomized controlled trials (RCTs): an experimental design in which subjects are randomly assigned to the experimental group (which receives the treatment or intervention under investigation) or to the control group (which receives no treatment, or a placebo).

Schizophrenia: a term coined by Bleuler for what is probably a group of disorders rather than a single disorder which is characterized by disturbance of multiple psychological processes (language and communication, thought content, mood, affect, sense of self, relationship to the external world, volition and motor behaviour). There has been considerable debate about the diagnostic criteria over the last few decades. However, within psychiatry, the criteria used in the *International Classification of Disease (ICD-10)* and the *Diagnostic and Statistical Manual of the American Psychiatric Association (DSM-IV)* are now generally applied in both clinical care and research.

Schizophrenogenic family: now considered to be an obsolete and discredited term but once used to describe a family (or specifically, mother) which was thought to have produced or fostered the development of schizophrenia in the child.

Service user: modern term for a person who uses psychiatric services. Alternative terms (patient, consumer) are still debated.

SSRIs (Selective Serotonin Reuptake Inhibitors): modern anti-depressants which act specifically on the serotonin neurotransmission system in the brain which is thought to be of key importance in the genesis of depression.

REFERENCES

Adams, G. and Cook, M. (1984) 'Beginning psychiatry', *Bulletin of the Royal College of Psychiatrists*, 8: 53–4.

Adshead, G. (1999) 'Duties of psychiatrists: treat the patient or protect the public?' *Advances in Psychiatric Treatment*, 5: 321–8.

Aitken, P., Perahia, D. and Wright, P. (2003) 'Psychiatrists entering the pharmaceutical industry in the UK', *Psychiatric Bulletin*, 27: 248–50.

Andreasen, N. (2001) *Brave New Brain: Conquering Mental Illness in the Era of the Genome*. New York: Oxford University Press.

Andrews, G. (2000) 'Meeting the unmet need with disease management', in G. Andrews and S. Henderson (eds), *Unmet Need in Psychiatry*. Cambridge: Cambridge University Press.

Arranz, M.J., Collier, D. and Kerwin, R.W. (2001) 'Pharmacogenetics for the individualization of psychiatric treatment', *American Journal of Pharmacogenomics*, 1: 3–10.

Arscott, K.J. (1999) 'ECT: the facts psychiatry declines to mention', in C. Newnes, G. Holmes and C. Dunn (eds), *This is Madness*. Ross-on-Wye: PCCS Books.

Artaud, A. (1947) 'Van Gogh, the man suicided by society', in S. Sontag (ed.), *Selected Works* (1988). Berkeley: University of California Press.

Baker, M.G., Kale, R., and Menken, M. (2002) 'The wall between neurology and psychiatry', *British Medical Journal*, 324: 1468–9.

Balint, M. (1964) *The Doctor, his Patient and the Illness*. London: Pitman.

Barker, P. (1992) *Regeneration*. Harmondsworth: Penguin.

Barnes, M. and Berke, J. (1991) *Two Accounts of a Journey Through Madness*. London: Free Association Books.

Battie, W.A. (1758) *Treatise on Madness*. London: Whiston.

Bayer, R. (1981) *Homosexuality and American Psychiatry: The Politics of Diagnosis*. New York: Basic Books.

Beck, A.T. (1976) *Cognitive Therapy and the Emotional Disorders*. New York: International Universities Press.

Bennet, G. (1979) *Patients and Their Doctors: The Journey through Medical Care*. London: Ballière Tindall.

Bennett, C. (2000) 'No shrinking violet: Raj Persaud, a psychiatrist for every occasion', *Guardian*, 31 August: 5.

Bennett, D.H. and Freeman, H.L. (1991) 'Principles and prospect', in D.L. Bennett and H.L. Freeman (eds), *Community Psychiatry: the Principles*. Edinburgh: Churchill Livingstone.

Bentall, R. (2003) *Madness Explained*. Harmondsworth: Penguin.

Beveridge, A. (1995) 'Madness in Victorian England: a study of patients admitted to the Royal Edinburgh Asylum under Thomas Clouston 1973–1908', *History of Psychiatry*, 16: 21–55.

Beveridge, A. (1998) 'R.D. Laing revisited', *Psychiatric Bulletin*, 22: 452–6.

Beveridge, A. (1999) 'The detective, the psychiatrists and post-modernism', *Psychiatric Bulletin*, 22: 573–4.

Bewley, T. (1998) 'Psychiatric Fellows of the Royal Society', *Psychiatric Bulletin*, 22: 377–80.

Bhugra, D. (1996) 'Religion and mental health', in D. Bhugra (ed.), *Psychiatry and Religion: Context, Consensus and Controversies*. London: Routledge.

Bhugra, D. and Cochrane, R. (eds) (2001) *Psychiatry in Multicultural Britain*. London: Gaskell.

Birchwood, M. (1991) 'Prescribing by psychologists?' *Psychiatric Bulletin*, 15: 34–5.

Blacker, C.P. (1946) *Neurosis in the Mental Health Services*. London: Oxford University Press.

Boyle, M. (1999) 'Diagnosis', in C. Newnes, G. Holmes and C. Dunn (eds), *This is Madness*. Ross-on-Wye: PCCS Books.

Bracken, P. (2002) 'Depression, psychiatry and the use of ECT', *Asylum*, 12: 26–8.

Bracken, P. and Thomas, P. (2001) 'Postpsychiatry: a new direction for mental health', *British Medical Journal*, 322: 724–7.

Breggin, P. (1993) *Toxic Psychiatry: Drugs and Electroconvulsive Therapy – the Truth and the Better Alternatives*. London: HarperCollins.

Brown, B. and Crawford, P. (2003) 'The clinical governance of the soul: "deep management" and the self-regulating subject in integrated community mental health teams', *Social Science and Medicine*, 56: 67–81.

Brown, P. (1999) 'Pierre Janet (1959–1947)', in H. Freeman (ed.), *A Century of Psychiatry*. London: Mosby.

Bruggen, P. (1997) *Who Cares: True Stories of the NHS Reforms*. Charlbury: Jon Carpenter.

Campbell, P. (1996) 'The history of the user movement in the United Kingdom', in T. Heller, J. Reynolds, R. Gomm et al. (eds), *Mental Health Matters: A Reader*. Basingstoke: Macmillan.

Campbell, R.J. (1989) *Psychiatric Dictionary* (6th Edition). New York: Oxford University Press.

Caplan, G. (1964) *Principles of Preventive Psychiatry*. London: Tavistock.

Carlsson, A. (1996) 'The rise of neuropsychopharmacology: impact on basic and clinical neuroscience', in D. Healy (ed.), *The Psychopharmacologists*, vol. 1. London: Arnold.

Castel, R. (1991) 'From dangerousness to risk', in G. Burchell, C. Gordon and P. Miller (eds), *The Foucault Effect: Studies in Governmentality*. Chicago: University of Chicago Press. pp. 281–98.

Castel, R., Castel, F. and Lovell, A. (1982) *The Psychiatric Society* (trans. from the French by A. Goldhammer), New York: Columbia University Press.

Cawthra, R. and Gibb, R. (1998) 'Severe personality disorder – whose responsibility?' *British Journal of Psychiatry*, 173: 8–10.

Chiswick, D. (1999) 'Prevention and detection – exhumed and enhanced', *Psychiatric Bulletin*, 23: 703–4.

Chiswick, D. (2001) 'Dangerous severe personality disorder – from notion to law', *Psychiatric Bulletin*, 25: 282–3.

Clare, A. (1980) *Psychiatry in Dissent: Controversial Issues in Thought and Practice* (2nd edition). London: Tavistock.

Clare, A. (1999) 'Democratic definitely, parochial possibly, challenged certainly: the College at the century's end', *Psychiatric Bulletin*, 23: 1–2.

Clark, D. (1985) Interviewed by Brian Baraclough. In G. Wilkinson (ed.) (1993) *Talking About Psychiatry*. London: Gaskell.

Clay, J. (1996) *R.D. Laing: A Divided Self*. London: Sceptre.

Connolly, K. (2002) 'Nazi Ghost Remains over Child Graves', *Guardian*, 29 April.

Cottrell, D. (1999) 'Recruitment, undergraduate education and the impact of *Tomorrow's Doctors*', *Psychiatric Bulletin*, 23: 582–4.

Cox, J., Marks, M., Marteau, L. and Steiner, J. (1982) 'Personal psychotherapy in the training of a psychiatrist', *Bulletin of the Royal College of Psychiatrists*, 6: 38–42.

Crane, H. (2003) 'Depression' (interview with Mike Shooter), *British Medical Journal*, 326: 1324–5.

Craven, M.A. and Bland, R. (eds) (2002) 'Shared mental health care: a bibliography and overview', *Canadian Journal of Psychiatry*, 47, Suppl. 1: 1–103S.

Creed, F. and Goldberg, D. (1987) 'Doctors' interest in psychiatry as a career', *Medical Education*, 21: 235–43.

Cullivan, R., Rooney, S., Kelly, G. and Walsh, N. (1999) 'Performance in psychiatry undergraduate finals: the influence of gender and nationality', *Psychiatric Bulletin*, 23: 280–2.

Deahl, M. (2002) 'Commentary: the alleged abuses of human rights in Chinese psychiatry', *Psychiatric Bulletin*, 26: 445–6.

Deahl, M. and Turner, T. (1997) 'General psychiatry in no-man's land', *British Journal of Psychiatry*, 171: 6–8.

Dean, A. (2001) *The Consultant Psychiatrist in the New Millennium*. London: Royal College of Psychiatrists.

Department of Health (1990) *The Care Programme Approach for People with a Mental Illness Referred to Specialist Psychiatric Services*, HC(90)23. London: HMSO.

Department of Health (2000) *The NHS Plan*. London: HMSO.

Department of Health and Department of Education (1991) *Working Together: Under the Children Act 1989*. London: HMSO.

Detre, T. and McDonald, M.C. (1997) 'Managed care and the future of psychiatry', *Archives of General Psychiatry*, 54: 201–4.

Dewar, I.G., Eagles, J.M., Klein, S., Gray, N. and Alexander, D.A. (2000) 'Psychiatric trainees' experiences of and reaction to patient suicide', *Psychiatric Bulletin*, 24: 20–23.

Double, D.B. (2001) 'Integrating critical psychiatry into psychiatric training', in C. Newnes, G. Holmes and C. Dunn (eds), *This is Madness Too*. Ross-on-Wye: PCCS Books.

Double, D. (2002) 'The limits of psychiatry', *British Medical Journal*, 324: 900–4.

Eisenberg, L. (1986) 'Mindlessness and brainlessness in psychiatry', *British Journal of Psychiatry*, 148: 497–508.

Eisenberg, L. (2000) 'Is psychiatry more mindful or brainier that it was a decade ago?' *British Journal of Psychiatry*, 176: 1–5.

Ellis, J. (1963) 'The teaching of psychiatry', *British Medical Journal*, 2: 585–8.

Engel, G. (1980) 'The clinical application of the biopsychosocial model', *American Journal of Psychiatry*, 137: 535–44.

Engstrom, E.J. and Weber, M.M. (1999) 'Emil Kraepelin (1856–1926)', in H. Freeman (ed.), *A Century of Psychiatry*. London: Mosby.

Eysenck, H.J. (1952) 'The effects of psychotherapy: an evaluation', *Journal of Consulting Psychology*, 16: 319–24.

Fernando, S. (1988) *Race and Culture in Psychiatry*. London: Croom Helm.

Finlayson, J. (1987) 'Political abuse of psychiatry with a special focus on the USSR: Report of a meeting held at the Royal College of Psychiatrists on 18 November 1986', *Bulletin of the Royal College of Psychiatrists*, 11: 144–5.

Firth-Cozens, J., Lema, V.C. and Firth, R.A. (1999) 'Specialty choice, stress and personality: their relationship over time', *Hospital Medicine*, 60: 751–5.

Fisher, S. (1996) 'Hanky-panky in the pharmaceutical industry', *International Journal of Psychopathology, Psychopharmacology and Psychotherapy*, 1 (URL http://www.psychcom.net/fisher.html).

Foucault, M. (1965) *Madness and Civilization: A History of Insanity in the Age of Reason*. London: Routledge.

Foucault, M. (1972) *The Archaeology of Knowledge* (translated from the French by A.M. Sheridan Smith). New York: Pantheon.

Foxton, M. (2002a) 'Bedside Stories', *Guardian*, 11 April.

Foxton, M. (2002b) 'Bedside Stories', *Guardian*, 9 May.

Frank, A.W. (1996) *The Wounded Storyteller: Body, Illness and Ethics*. Chicago: University of Chicago Press.

Freud, S. (1900) *The Interpretation of Dreams* (translated from the German by A.A. Brill in 1913). New York: Macmillan.

Freud, S. (1901) *The Psychopathology of Everyday Life* (translated from the German by A.A. Brill in 1914). London: T. Fisher Unwin.

Fulford, K.W.M. (1996) 'Religion and psychiatry: extending the limits of tolerance in Religion and mental health', in D. Bhugra (ed.), *Psychiatry and Religion: Context, Consensus and Controversies*. London: Routledge.

Fulford, K.W.M., Morris, K.J., Sadler, J.Z. and Stanghellini, G. (2003) 'Past improbable, future, possible: the renaissance in philosophy and psychiatry', in K.W.M. Fulford, K.J. Morris, J.Z. Sadler, and G. Stanghellini (eds), *Nature and Narrative: An Introduction to the New Philosophy of Psychiatry*. Oxford: Oxford University Press.

Gask, L. (1997) 'Listening to patients' (Editorial), *British Journal of Psychiatry*, 17: 301–2.

Gask, L. and McGrath, G. (1989) 'Psychotherapy and general practice: a review', *British Journal of Psychiatry*, 154: 445–53.

Gask, L., Sibbald, B. and Creed, F. (1997) 'Evaluating models of working at the interface between mental health services and primary care', *British Journal of Psychiatry*, 170: 6–11.

Gask, L., Rogers, A., Oliver, D., May, C. and Roland, M. (2003) 'Qualitative study of patients' views of the quality of care for depression in general practice', *British Journal of General Practice*, 53: 278–83.

Gater, R., de Almeida e Sousa, B., Barrientos, G., Caraveo, J., Chandrashekar, C.R., Dhadphale, M., Goldberg, D., Al Kathiri, A.H., Mubbashar, M., Silhan, K., Thong, D., Torees-Gonzales, F. and Sartorius, N. (1991) 'The pathways to psychiatric care: a cross-cultural study', *Psychological Medicine*, 21: 761–74.

Geddes, J. (1998) 'Evidence-based psychiatry: a practical approach', *Psychiatric Bulletin*, 22: 337–8.

Gelder, M.G. (1991) 'Aldolf Meyer', in G.E. Berrios and H. Freeman (eds), *150 Years of British Psychiatry*, vol 1. London: Gaskell.

General Medical Council (1995) *Guidance to Doctors*. London: GMC.

Goffman, E. (1961) *Asylums: Essays on the Social Situation of Mental Patients*. New York: Doubleday.

Goldberg, D. and Gournay, K. (1997) 'The general practitioner, the psychiatrist and the burden of mental health care', *Maudsley Discussion Paper no: 1*. London: Institute of Psychiatry.

Goldberg, D. and Murray, R. (eds) (2002) *The Maudsley Handbook of Practical Psychiatry* (4th edition). Oxford: Oxford University Press.

Goldman, W. (2001) 'Is there a shortage of psychiatrists?' *Psychiatric Services*, 52: 1587–9.

Greenberg, M., Szmukler, G. and Tantam, D. (1986) *Making Sense of Psychiatric Cases*. Oxford: Oxford University Press.

Greenhalgh, T. and Hurwitz, B. (1998) 'Why study narrative?' in T. Greenhalgh and B. Hurwitz (eds), *Narrative Based Medicine*. London: BMJ Books.

Guthrie, E. and Black, D. (1997) 'Psychiatric disorder, stress and burnout', *Advances in Psychiatric Treatment*, 3: 275–81.

Hacking, I. (1995) *Rewriting the Soul: Multiple Personality and the Science of Memory.* Princeton, NJ: Princeton University Press.

Haigh, R. (2000) 'Support systems. 2. Staff sensitivity groups', *Advances in Psychiatric Treatment*, 6: 312–19.

Hart, D. (2001) 'Memoirs of a press officer', *Psychiatric Bulletin*, 5: 189–90.

Hawton, K., Clements, A., Sakarovitch, C., Simkin, S. and Deeks, J.S. (2001) 'Suicide in doctors: a study of risk according to gender, seniority and speciality in medical practitioners in England and Wales, 1979–1995', *Journal of Epidemiology and Community Health*, 55: 296–300.

Healy, D. (1997) *The Antidepressant Era.* Boston: Harvard.

Healy, D. (2000) 'A dance to the music of the century', *Psychiatric Bulletin*, 24: 1–3.

Healy, D. (2001) 'Evidence biased psychiatry', *Psychiatric Bulletin*, 25: 290–1.

Hervey, N. (1985) 'A slavish bowing down: the Lunacy Commission and the psychiatric Profession 1945–60', in Bynum, W.F., Porter, R. and Shepherd, M. (eds), *The Anatomy of Madness*, vol. II: *Institutions and Society.* London: Tavistock.

Hiroch, U. Appleby, L., Mortensen, P.B. and Dunn, G. (2001) 'Death by homicide, suicide and other unnatural causes in people with mental illness: a population-based study', *Lancet*, 358: 2110–12.

Hobson, J.A. and Leonard, J. (2001) *Out of its Mind: Psychiatry in Crisis – a Call for Reform.* Cambridge, Mass.: Perseus Publishing.

Holloway, F. (1999) 'The College: a leadership role in mental health services?' *Psychiatric Bulletin*, 23: 324–5. Invited commentary on R.E. Kendell, 'Influencing The Department of Health', in ibid.: 321–3.

Holmes, G. and Dunn, C. (1999) Introduction to *This is Madness: A Critical Look at Psychiatry and the Future of Mental Health Services*, (ed.) by C. Newnes, G. Holmes and C. Dunn. Ross-on-Wye: PCCS Books.

Holmes, J. (2000) 'Fitting together the biopsychosocial jigsaw', *British Journal of Psychiatry*, 177: 93–4.

Horowitz, A.V. (2002) *Creating Mental Illness.* Chicago: University of Chicago Press.

Hunter, R. and MacAlpine, I. (1963) *Three Hundred Years of Psychiatry, 1535–1860.* London: Oxford University Press.

James, W. (1977) *The Varieties of Religious Experience: A Study in Human Nature.* Glasgow: Collins.

Jaspers, K. (1913) *General Psychopathology* (7th edition), 1959 (translated by J. Hoenig and M.W. Hamilton. Manchester: Manchester University Press).

Jenkins, R., McCulloch, A., Friedli, L. and Parker, C. (2002) *Developing a National Mental Health Policy.* Hove: Psychology Press.

Johnstone, L. (2000) *Users and Abusers of Psychiatry* (2nd edition). London: Brunner-Routledge.

Jones, E. (1959) *Free Associations.* New York: Basic Books.

Jones, H. (1994) 'All theory, no understanding', *Openmind*, 69: 6.

Jones, K. (1993) *Asylums and After.* London: Athlone.

Jones, K.S. (1998) 'The other end of the couch', *Psychiatric Bulletin*, 22: 515–16.

Jones, M. (1983) Interview by Brian Baraclough, in E. Wilkinson (ed.) (1993), *Talking About Psychiatry.* London: Gaskell.

Katon, W., Robinson, P., Von Korff, M., Lin, E., Bush, T., Ludman, E., Simon, G. and Walker, E. (1996) 'A multifaceted intervention to improve treatment of depression in primary care', *Archives of General Psychiatry*, 53: 924–32.

Kelly, B.D. and McLoughlin, D.M. (2002) 'Euthanasia, assisted suicide and psychiatry: a Pandora's box', British Journal of Psychiatry, 181: 278–9.

Kendell, R.E. (1975) *The Role of Diagnosis in Psychiatry.* Oxford: Blackwell.

Kendell, R.E. (1998) 'What are Royal Colleges for?' *Psychiatric Bulletin*, 22: 721–3.
Kendell, R.E. (1999) 'Influencing the Department of Health', *Psychiatric Bulletin*, 23: 321–3.
Kendell, R.E. (2000) 'The next 25 years', *British Journal of Psychiatry*, 176: 6–9.
Kendell, R. and Pearce, A. (1997) 'Consultant psychiatrists who retired prematurely in 1995 and 1996', *Psychiatric Bulletin*, 21: 741–54.
Kendell, R.E., Cooper, J.E. and Gourley, A.J. (1971) 'Diagnostic criteria of American and British Psychiatrists', *Archives of General Psychiatry*, 25: 123–30.
Kennedy, P. (2000) 'Is psychiatry losing touch with the rest of medicine?' *Advances in Psychiatric Treatment*, 6: 16–21.
Kennedy, P. and Griffiths, H. (2001) 'General psychiatrists discovering new roles for a new era ... and removing work stress', *British Journal of Psychiatry*, 179: 283–5.
Kennedy, P. and Griffiths, H. (2002) 'What does "responsible medical officer" mean in a modern mental health service?', *Psychiatric Bulletin*, 26: 205–8.
Kessel, N. (1963) 'Who ought to see a psychiatrist?' *Lancet*, 1: 1092–5.
Kessel, N. (1996) 'Should we buy liaison psychiatry?', *Journal of the Royal Society of Medicine*, 89: 481–2.
Kleinman, A. (1991) *Rethinking Psychiatry: from Cultural Category to Personal Experience.* New York: Free Press.
Kohen, D. and Arnold, E. (2002) 'The female psychiatrist: professional, personal and social issues', *Advances in Psychiatric Treatment*, 8: 81–8.
Kraus, A. (2003) 'How can the phenomenological–anthropological approach contribute to diagnosis and classification in psychiatry?', in K.W.M. Fulford, K.J. Morris, J.Z. Sadler and G. Stanghellini (eds), *Nature and Narrative: An Introduction to the New Philosophy of Psychiatry.* Oxford: Oxford University Press.
Laing, R.D. (1960) *The Divided Self.* London: Tavistock.
Laugharne, R. (1999) 'Evidence-based medicine, user involvement and the post-modern paradigm', *Psychiatric Bulletin*, 23: 641–3.
Laurance, J. (2003) *Pure Madness: How Fear Drives the Mental Health System.* London: Routledge.
Lewis, A. (1950) 'Henry Maudsley: his work and influence', in A. Lewis, *The State of Psychiatry: Essays and Addresses* (1967). London: Routledge.
Lewis, A.J. (1955) 'Health as a social concept', *British Journal of Sociology*, 4: 109–24.
Lipsedge, M. (1996) 'Religion and madness in history', in D. Bhugra (ed.), *Psychiatry and Religion: Context, Consensus and Controversies.* London: Routledge.
Littlejohns, C.S., Wilkinson, G. and Murphy, E. (1992) 'Training psychiatrists for work in the community', *Psychiatric Bulletin*, 16: 23–4.
Littlewood, R. (1996) 'Psychiatry's culture', *International Journal of Social Psychiatry*, 42: 245–65.
Littlewood, R. and Lipsedge, R. (1997) *Aliens and Alienists: Ethnic Minorities and Psychiatry* (3rd edition). London: Routledge.
Lott, T. (1996) *The Scent of Dried Roses.* London: Viking.
Luhrmann, T.M. (2000) *Of Two Minds: The Growing Disorder in American Psychiatry.* New York: Alfred A. Knopf.
Lyons, D. and O'Malley, A. (2002) 'The labelling of dissent: politics and psychiatry behind the Great Wall', *Psychiatric Bulletin*, 26: 434–4.
Madden, J.S. (2000) 'Euthanasia in Nazi Germany', *Psychiatric Bulletin*, 24: 347.
Maden, T. (1999) 'Treating offenders with personality disorder', *Psychiatric Bulletin*, 23: 707–10.
Main, T. (1946) 'The hospital as a therapeutic institution', *Bulletin of the Menninger Clinic*, 10: 66–71.

Makinson, J. (1973) *The story of Whittington Hospital 1873–1973*. Preston: Whittington Hospital Management Committee.

Masson, J.M. (1992) *The Assault on Truth: Freud and Child Sexual Abuse*. New York: HarperPerennial.

Mathers, N. and Hodgkin, P. (1989) 'The gatekeeper and the wizard: a fairytale', *British Medical Journal*, 298: 172–3.

May, C., Gask, L., Atkinson, T., Ellis, N., Mair, F. and Esmail, A. (2001) 'Resisting and promoting new technologies in clinical practice: the case of telepsychiatry', *Social Science and Medicine*, 52: 1889–901.

Mayou, R. (1997) 'Psychiatry, medicine and consultation–liaison', *British Journal of Psychiatry*, 171: 203–4.

McCready, J.R. and Waring, E.M. (1986) 'Interviewing skills in relation to psychiatric residency', *Canadian Journal of Psychiatry*, 31: 317–32.

McGrath, P. (1997) *Asylum*. Harmondsworth: Penguin.

McHugh, P. and Slavney, P.R. (1998) *The Perspectives of Psychiatry* (2nd edition). Baltimore: Johns Hopkins University Press.

McIvor, R. (2001) 'Care and compulsion in community psychiatric treatment', *Psychiatric Bulletin*, 25: 369–70.

McKenzie, K. (1998) 'Autonomy and automatons: managed care in the USA', *Psychiatric Bulletin*, 22: 765–8.

Mechanic, D. (1999a) *Mental Health and Social Policy: The Emergence of Managed Care*. Needham Heights, MA: Allyn & Bacon.

Mechanic, D. (1999b) 'Definitions and perspectives', in A.V. Horowitz and T.L. Scheid (eds), *A Handbook for the Study of Mental Health*. Cambridge: Cambridge University Press.

Mental Health Foundation (2000) *Strategies for Living: The Research Report*. London: Mental Health Foundation.

Meyer, A. (1952) *The Collected Papers of Adolf Meyer*. Baltimore: Johns Hopkins University Press.

Meyer, A. (1956) *Psychobiology: A Science of Man*. Springfield, IL: C.C. Thomas.

Moniz, E. (1927) 'Pre-frontal leucotomy in the treatment of mental disorder', *American Journal of Psychiatry*, 93: 1379–85.

Montague, L. (1990) 'The psychiatrist in the community mental health team', *Psychiatric Bulletin*, 14: 19–20.

Morel, B.-A. (1857) *Traité des dégénérescences*. Paris: Baillière.

Morris, D.B. (2000) *Illness and Culture in the Postmodern Age*. Berkeley and Los Angeles: University of California Press.

Mosher, L.R. (1999) 'I want no part of it anymore', *Psychology Today*, 32: 2–4.

Mubbashar, M.H. and Humayun, A. (1999) 'Training psychiatrists in Britain to work in developing countries', *Advances in Psychiatric Treatment*, 5: 443–6.

Munro, R. (2002) *Dangerous Minds: Political Psychiatry in China today and its Origins in the Mao Era*. New York/Hilversum: Human Rights Watch and Geneva Initiative on Psychiatry.

Murray, C.J.L and Lopez, A.D. (eds) (1995) *The Global Burden of Disease*. Cambridge, MA: Harvard University Press.

Neelerman, J. and van Os, J. (1994) 'The feasibility of a psychiatric common-market', *Psychiatric Bulletin*, 18: 193–5.

Nelson, S.H. and Torrey, E.F. (1973) 'The religious functions of psychiatry', *American Jounal of Orthopsychiatry*, 43: 362–7.

Newnes, C. (1999) 'Histories of psychiatry', in C. Newnes, G. Holmes and C. Dunn (eds), *This is Madness*. Ross-on-Wye: PCCS Books.

NHS Executive (1996) *NHS Psychotherapy Services in England: Review of Strategic Policy*. London: Department of Health.

NHSE (1999) *National Service Framework for Mental Health*. London: HMSO.

Owen, J. (1992) 'Death threats to psychiatrists', *Psychiatric Bulletin*, 16: 142–4.

Peck, E., Gulliver, P. and Towel, D. (2002) 'Information, consultation or control: user involvement in mental health services in England at the turn of the century', *Journal of Mental Health*, 11: 441–51.

Perinpanayagam, M.S. (1973) 'Overseas psychiatric doctors', News and Notes Supplement. *British Journal of Psychiatry*, cited in A. Clare. (1980) *Psychiatry in Dissent Controversial Issues in Thought and Practice* (2nd edition). London: Tavistock.

Persaud, R. (2000a) 'Psychiatry in the new millennium', *Psychiatric Bulletin*, 24: 16–19.

Persaud, R. (2000b) 'Psychiatrists suffer from stigma too', *Psychiatric Bulletin*, 24: 284–5.

Persaud, R. and Meux, C.J. (1990) 'Clinical examination for professional qualification in psychiatry: the patients' views', *Psychiatric Bulletin*, 14: 65–71.

Peters, U.W. (1999) 'German Psychiatry', in H. Freeman (ed.), *A Century of Psychiatry*. London: Mosby.

Pilgrim, D. (2002) 'The biopsychosocial model in Anglo-American psychiatry: past, present and future?' *Journal of Mental Health*, 11: 585–94.

Pilgrim, D. and Rogers, A. (1993) *A Sociology of Mental Health and Illness*. Buckingham: Open University Press.

Pincus, H.A., Zarin, D.A., Tanieilan, T.L., Johnson, J.L., West, J.C., Petit, A.R., Marcus, S.C., Kessler, R.C. and McIntyre, J.S. (1999) 'Psychiatric patients and treatments in 1997', *Archives of General Psychiatry*, 56: 441–9.

Pippard, J. and Ellam, L. (1981) 'Electroconvulsive treatment in Britain', *British Journal of Psychiatry*, 139: 563–8.

Plath, S. (1963) *The Bell Jar*. London: Heinemann.

Porter, R. (2002) *Madness: A Brief History*. Oxford: Oxford University Press.

Pullen, I.M. and Yellowlees, A.J. (1988) 'Scottish psychiatrists in primary health-care settings: a silent majority', *British Journal of Psychiatry*, 153: 663–6.

Rees, H., Sipos, A., Spence, M. and Harrison, G. (2002) 'Attitudes of psychiatrists to evidence-based guidelines: a questionnaire survey', *Psychiatric Bulletin*, 26: 421–4.

Rees, W.L. (1952) 'A comparative study of the value of insulin coma, electronarcosis, electroshock and leucotomy', in the *Treatment of Schizophrenia. Premier Congrès Mondial de Psychiatrie, Paris, 1950, vol 4: Thérapeutique Biologique*. Paris: Hermann, pp. 303–8.

Ring, H., Mumford, D. and Katona, C. (1999) 'Psychiatry in the new undergraduate curriculum', *Advances in Psychiatric Treatment*, 5: 415–9.

Rippere, V. and Williams, R. (1985) *Wounded Healers: Mental Health Workers' Experiences of Depression*. Chichester: Wiley.

Ritchie, J.H., Dick, D. and Lingham, R. (1994) *The Report of the Inquiry into the Care and Treatment of Christopher Clunis*. London: HMSO.

Roach, J. and Dorling, D. (2000) 'Recruiting the wrong students', *Student British Medical Journal*, 8: 178–9.

Roberts, G.A. (2000) 'Narratives and severe mental illness: what place do stories have in an evidence-based world?' *Advances in Psychiatric Treatment*, 6: 432–41.

Robertson, J.A. (1994) 'Community psychiatry. Weasel words? A personal view', *Psychiatric Bulletin*, 18: 760–1.

Rogers, A., Pilgrim, D. and Lacey, R. (1993) *Experiencing Psychiatry: Users' Views of Services*. Basingstoke: Macmillan/MIND.

Rogler, L.H. (1997) 'Making sense of historical changes in the *Diagnostic and Statistical Manual of Mental Disorders:* Five propositions', *Journal of Health and Social Behaviour,* 38: 9–20.

Rogow, A.A. (1970) *The Psychiatrists.* New York: Delta.

Romano, J. (1994) 'Reminiscences: 1938 and since', *American Journal of Psychiatry,* 151 (Sesquicentennial Suppl.): 83–9.

Rose, D., Fleischmann, P., Wykes, T., Leese, M. and Bindman, J. (2003) 'Patients' perspectives on electroconvulsive therapy: systematic review', *British Medical Journal,* 326: 1363–7.

Rose, N. (1996) 'Psychiatry as a political science: advanced liberalism and the administration of risk', *History of the Human Sciences,* 9: 1–23.

Rosenhan, D.L. (1973) 'On being sane in insane places', *Science,* 179: 250–8.

Rowe, D. (1993) 'Foreword', in P. Breggin, *Toxic Psychiatry: Drugs and Electroconvulsive Therapy: The Truth and the Better Alternatives.* London: HarperCollins.

Royal College of Psychiatrists (1995) *The ECT Handbook (Second Report of the Royal College of Psychiatrists' Special Committee on ECT),* Council Report CR39. London: Royal College of Psychiatrists.

Royal College of Psychiatrists (1996) *The Responsibilities of Consultant Psychiatrists.* Revised statement. Council Report CRSI. London: Royal College of Psychiatrists.

Royal College of Psychiatrists (1999) *Guidelines for Healthcare Commissioners for an ECT Service,* Royal College of Psychiatrists' Special Committee on ECT, Council Report CR73. London: Royal College of Psychiatrists.

Royal College of Psychiatrists (2001) *Role and Contribution of the Consultant Psychiatrist in Psychotherapy in the NHS.* Council Report CR98. London: Royal College of Psychiatrists.

Royal College of Psychiatrists (2002) *Annual Census of Psychiatric Staffing 2001.* Occasional paper OP54. London: Royal College of Psychiatrists.

Rutter, D. and Cox, A. (1981) 'Psychiatric interviewing techniques: I. Methods and Measures', *British Journal of Psychiatry,* 138: 273–82.

Sabin, J.E. (1995) 'Organised psychiatry and managed care: quality improvement or holy war?' *Health Affairs* (Fall): 32–3.

Sartorius, N. (2002) *Fighting for Mental Health: A Personal View.* Cambridge: Cambridge University Press.

Sartorius, N., Jablensky, A., Korten, A., Ernberg, G., Anker, M., Cooper, J.E. and Day, R. (1986) 'Early manifestations and first contact incidence of schizophrenia in different cultures', *Psychological Medicine,* 7: 529–41.

Scally, G. and Donaldson, L.J. (1998) 'Clinical governance and the drive for quality improvement in the new NHS in England', *British Medical Journal,* 317: 61–5.

Schlesinger, M., Dorwat, R.A. and Epstein, S.S. (1996) 'Managed care constraints on psychiatrists' hospital practices: bargaining power and professional autonomy', *American Journal of Psychiatry,* 153: 256–60.

Schneider, I. (1987) 'The theory and practice of movie psychiatry', *American Journal of Psychiatry,* 144: 996–1002.

Scott, J. (1986) 'What puts medical students off psychiatry?' *Bulletin of the Royal College of Psychiatrists,* 10: 98–100.

Scull, A. (1979) *Museums of Madness.* Harmondsworth: Penguin.

Scull, A. (1984) 'Was insanity increasing? A response to Edward Hare', *British Journal of Psychiatry,* 144: 432–6.

Sedgwick, P. (1982) *Psychopolitics.* London: Pluto.

Shaw, F. (1997) *Out of Me: The Story of a Postnatal Breakdown.* London: Viking.

Shea, S.C. (1998) *Psychiatric Interviewing: The Art of Understanding* (2nd edition). Philadelphia: Saunders.

Shepherd, B. (1999) 'Shell-Shock', in H. Freeman (ed.), *A Century of Psychiatry*. London: Mosby.

Shepherd, B. (2002) *A War of Nerves: Soldiers and Psychiatrists 1914–1994*. London: Pimlico.

Shepherd, M. (1976) 'Definition, classification and nomenclature: a clinical overview', in D. Kemali, G. Bartholini and D. Richer (eds), *Schizophrenia Today*. Oxford: Pergamon.

Shepherd, M. (1991) Interview by Greg Wilkinson, in G. Wilkinson (ed.) (1993), *Talking About Psychiatry*. London: Gaskell.

Shorter, E. (1997) *A History of Psychiatry: From the Era of the Asylum to the Age of Prozac*. New York: John Wiley.

Sierles, F.S. and Taylor, M.A. (1995) 'Decline of US medical student career choice of psychiatry and what to do about it', *American Journal of Psychiatry*, 152: 1416–26.

Sigal, C. (1976) *Zone of the Interior*. New York: Thomas Cromwell.

Simon, G. (1999) 'The contribution of psychiatrists to management in primary care', in M. Tansella and G. Thornicroft (eds), *Common Disorders in Primary Care – Essays in Honour of Professor Sir David Goldberg*. London: Routledge.

Sims, A. (2003) *Symptoms in the Mind: An Introduction to Descriptive Pathology*. (3rd edition). Edinburgh: Saunders.

Stanton, M. (1999) 'The emergence of psychoanalysis', in H. Freeman (ed.), *A Century of Psychiatry*. London: Mosby.

Stevens, A. and Price, J. (2000) *Evolutionary Psychiatry: A New Beginning*. London: Routledge.

Storer, D. (1998) 'Too many patients; too few psychiatrists', *Psychiatric Bulletin*, 22: 724–5.

Storer, D. (2002) 'Recruiting and retaining psychiatrists', *British Journal of Psychiatry*, 180: 296–7.

Strathdee, G. and Williams, P. (1984) 'A survey of psychiatrists in primary care: the silent growth of a new service', *Journal of the Royal College of General Practitioners*, 34: 615–18.

Strickland, P.L., Deakin, J.F., Percival, C., Gater, R.A. and Goldberg, D. (2002) 'Biosocial origins of depression in the community: interaction between social adversity, cortisol and serotonin neurotransmission', *British Journal of Psychiatry*, 180: 168–73.

Styron, W. (1992) *Darkness Visible*. London: Picador.

Sutherland, S. (1995) *Breakdown: A Personal Crisis and a Medical Dilemma*. Oxford: Oxford University Press.

Szasz, T.S. (1974) *The Myth of Mental Illness*. New York: Harper and Row.

Szatmari, P. (1999) 'Evidence based child psychiatry and the two solitudes', *Evidence Based Mental Health*, 2: 6–7.

Szmukler, G. (2000) 'Homicide inquiries: what sense do they make?' *Psychiatric Bulletin*, 24: 6–10.

Talbott, J.A. and Hales, R.E. (2001) *Administrative Psychiatry: New Concepts for a Changing Behavioral Health System* (2nd edition). Washington, DC. American Psychiatric Publishing, Inc.

Tansella, M. (2001) 'The psychiatrist as archaeologist and architect', *Advances in Psychiatric Treatment*, 7: 81–2.

Tantam, D. (1991) 'The Anti-Psychiatry Movement', in G.E. Berrios and H.L. Freeman (eds), *150 Years of British Psychiatry*, vol 1. London: Gaskell.

Tantam, D., Appleby, L. and Duncan, A. (1996) *Psychiatry for the Developing World*. London: Gaskell.

Tarasoff v. Regents of the University of California et al. 131 Cal Rpt 14, 551, P2d34 (Cal 1976).

Temple, N. (1999) 'Should consultant psychiatrists be trained in psychotherapy?' *Advances in Psychiatric Treatment*, 5: 288–95.

Thomas, K. (1971) *Religion and the Decline of Magic*. London: Penguin.

Thomas, P.F. and Bracken, P. (1999) 'The value of advocacy: putting ethics into practice', *Psychiatric Bulletin*, 23: 327–9.

Thompson, C. (1998) 'The mental state we are in: morale and psychiatry', *Psychiatric Bulletin*, 22: 405–9.

Thornicroft, G. and Goldberg, D. (1998) *Has Community Care Failed?* Maudsley Discussion Paper No. 5. London: Maudsley Hospital.

Timms, P. (2003) 'The consultant psychiatrists – a remembrance of things past?' *Psychiatric Bulletin*, 27: 47–9.

Toone, B.K., Murray, R., Clare, A., Creed, F. and Smith, A. (1979) 'Psychiatrists' models of mental illness and their personal backgrounds', *Psychological Medicine*, 9: 165–78.

Tooth, G.C. and Brooke, E.M. (1961) 'Trends in the mental hospital population and their effect on future planning', *Lancet*, i: 710–13.

Tredgold, R.F. and Wolff, H.H. (1975) *University College Hospital Notes on Psychiatry*. London: Duckworth.

Turner, T.H. (1989) 'Schizophrenia and mental handicap: an historical review with implications for further research', *Psychological Medicine*, 19: 301–14.

Turner, T.H. (1999) 'The Early 1900s and before...', in H. Freeman (ed.), *A Century of Psychiatry*. London: Mosby.

Turner, T., Salter, M. and Deahl, M. (1999) 'Mental Health Act reform: should psychiatrists go on being responsible?' *Psychiatric Bulletin*, 23: 578–81.

Tyrer, P. (1998) 'Whither community care?' *British Journal of Psychiatry*, 173: 359–60.

UK ECT Review Group (2003) 'Efficacy and safety of electroconvulsive therapy in depressive disorders: a systematic review and meta-analysis', *Lancet*, 361: 799–808.

Valenstein, E.S. (1986) *Great Hopes and Desperate Cures*. New York: Basic Books.

Valenstein, E.S. (1998) *Blaming the Brain*. New York: Free Press.

van Voren, R. (2002) 'The WPA World Congress in Yokohama and the issue of political abuse of psychiatry in China', *Psychiatric Bulletin*, 26: 441–2.

Wall, T.D., Bolden, R.I., Borrill, C.S., Carter, A.J., Golya, D.A., Hardy, G.E., Haynes, C.E., Rick, J.E., Shapiro, D.A. and West, M.A. (1997) 'Minor psychiatric disorder in NHS trust staff: occupational and gender differences', *British Journal of Psychiatry*, 171: 519–23.

Weir Mitchell, S. (1894) Address before the Fiftieth Annual Meeting of the American Medico-Psychological Association, Philadelphia, published in the *Journal of Nervous and Mental Diseases* (1894) 21: 413–37.

Weissman, S., Sabshin, M. and Eist, H. (1999) *Psychiatry in the New Millennium*. Washington, DC: American Psychiatric Press.

Wessely, S. (1996) 'The rise of counselling and the return of alienism', *British Medical Journal*, 313: 158–60.

Wessely, S. and Lutz, T. (1995) 'Neurasthenia', in G. Berrios and R. Porter (eds), *A History of Clinical Psychiatry*. London: Athlone.

WHO (1973) *Report of the International Pilot Study of Schizophrenia*. Geneva: World Health Organization.

WHO (2000) *World Health Organization Guide to Common Mental Disorders and Emotional Problems*. London: Royal Society of Medicine.

Wilkinson, D.G., Greer, S. and Toone, B. (1983) 'Medical students' attitudes to psychiatry', *Psychological Medicine*, 13: 185–92.

Williams, K. (1998) 'Self-assessment of clinical competence by general practitioner trainees before and after a six-month psychiatric placement', *British Journal of General Practice*, 48: 1387–90.

Wilson, M. (1993) 'DSM–III and the transformation of American Psychiatry', *American Journal of Psychiatry*, 150: 399–410.

Wolff, H. (1988) Interview by Sidney Bloch, in G. Wilkinson (ed.) (1993), *Talking About Psychiatry*. London: Gaskell.

Wootton, R., Yellowlees, P. and McLaren, P. (eds) (2003) *Telepsychiatry and E-Mental Health*. London: Royal Society of Medicine Press.

WPA (2002) *Institutional Program on the Core Training Curriculum for Psychiatry*. Yokohama: World Psychiatric Association.

WPA and WFME (1998) *Core Curriculum in Psychiatry for Medical Students*. New York: World Psychiatric Association and World Federation for Medical Education.

Wright, A.F. (1997) 'What a general practitioner can expect from a consultant psychiatrist', *Advances in Psychiatric Treatment*, 3: 25–31.

Wurtzel, E. (1995) *Prozac Nation: Young and Depressed in America*. London: Quartet.

INDEX

Page numbers in **bold** indicate a glossary entry